Living Well After Diagnosis

Practical Strategies to Cope, Move Forward, and Reclaim Your Life with Chronic Illness

Robert H. Phillips, Ph.D.

Internationally renowned psychologist & author

LIVING WELL AFTER DIAGNOSIS
Practical Strategies to Cope, Move Forward,
and Reclaim Your Life with Chronic Illness

Coping:

"Consistently, actively, and consciously using learned, specific strategies that can change the things you do or the way you think— so you can manage or control those specific factors, problems, situations, or circumstances that are current or potential obstacles to your happiness and well-being."

© *Robert H. Phillips, Ph.D.*

Living Well After Diagnosis

Proven Strategies to Cope, Move Forward, and Reclaim Your Life with Chronic Illness

Robert H. Phillips, Ph.D.

Table of Contents

Introduction

The diagnosis of a serious illness or condition is one of the scariest, most life-changing experiences a person can have. For some, it comes out of the blue. For others, it follows a long period of uncertainty, doctor visits, and unanswered questions.

No matter how it arrives, once a doctor utters the words, "You have [fill in the medical condition]," your life changes instantly. Suddenly, you are faced with new realities—medical, emotional, and practical. One of the most important things to remember in this moment is simple but powerful: never lose hope.

Of course, your diagnosis will affect you. You are human, and your world has been shaken. Not only may you feel different physically, but you also face adjustments in how you view yourself, how you manage symptoms and treatments, and how you navigate your daily routines.

This combination of practical changes and psychological challenges can be overwhelming. Yet, here is the good news: your life can still be good—sometimes even better—than before your diagnosis. How could that be possible? You'll see as you go through this book... and you'll learn what you can do to make this happen.

Although your physical condition may be altered, that doesn't mean you can't become healthier. The goal is to be as healthy as possible within the reality of your condition, while also enhancing the many other parts of your life that remain open to growth and fulfillment. Your aim is not just survival, but to reclaim your life and live it as fully as you can, even with a chronic illness.

So, you stand at a crossroads. You have two choices:

1. Allow your diagnosis to overwhelm you, leaving you feeling defeated and unable to do the things you value; or
2. Take the road of coping, growth, and positive action to regain control and improve your emotional well-being.

I believe you've chosen the second road—because you're reading this book. And this book can help!

Be Prepared

Living with chronic illness may affect you in countless ways. It can:

- Interfere with daily activities
- Change your physical functioning
- Lead to lifestyle adjustments
- Affect your emotions (causing depression, anxiety, anger, guilt, helplessness, and other feelings)
- Affect relationships with family and friends
- Alter your social life
- Disrupt work or career goals
- Cause appetite or weight changes
- Disturb your sleep
- Leave you feeling out of control

These are powerful reasons to take action—to learn how to cope and to put effective strategies in place.

What Kind of Book Is This?

This book is a "what to do" toolbox. It won't overwhelm you in lengthy case studies or complex academic language. Instead, it will take your hand and offer practical strategies you can begin using right now to start living well after your diagnosis.

The book focuses on workable suggestions—things you can implement immediately to ease stress, boost resilience, and move forward. You'll read about steps you can take right away to regain a sense of control. (Yes, it is possible!) You'll find tips, reminders, and strategies that support not only your health, but also your happiness, relationships, and productivity.

No single book can cover every possible strategy, but this one gives you a solid starting point—and a wide range of tools you can adapt to your own journey.

Two Main Goals

When living with chronic illness, you face two major challenges:

1. Doing what you can about the illness itself.
2. Coping with the many ways it affects your life.

This book will help with both—and, most importantly, it will guide you to achieve the ultimate goal: taking charge of your life and creating a future that feels meaningful, productive, and fulfilling.

How This Book Is Organized

Research shows that people who manage their diagnoses most successfully tend to:

- Learn as much as possible about their condition
- Partner with their healthcare team as informed patients
- Stay as active as possible

- Cultivate positive mental attitudes
- Regain control of their lives

This book is built around those principles. It is divided into 10 chapters, each focusing on one key area of coping and growth. Each chapter contains strategies, tips, and reminders tailored to that theme.

Here's a quick roadmap:

- **Chapter 1: I Need to Get Ready to Help Myself**—work on foundational strategies to prepare your mindset and create a strong base for coping.

- **Chapter 2: I Need to Understand What's Happening**—make sense of your diagnosis and the emotions that often come with it.

- **Chapter 3: I Need to Accept and Adapt** — learn how to grieve the loss of former health, embrace your "new normal," and prepare for what's to come

- **Chapter 4: I Need to Find My Pace and Priorities**---begin resuming daily life, rebuilding routines, and regaining momentum after the initial shock.

- **Chapter 5: I Need to Be an Active Treatment Partner**—stay actively engaged in your care and collaborate with your medical team.

- **Chapter 6: I Need to Get the Right Care from the Right People**—choose the right professionals and make the most of appointments and professional guidance.

- **Chapter 7: I Need to Strengthen My Mindset and Resilience**—benefit from tools to build resilience, a positive mindset, and emotional steadiness.

- **Chapter 8: I Need to Support My Body Wisely**—support your body with sustainable lifestyle and health-related strategies.

- **Chapter 9: I Need to Strengthen My Circle of Support**—make the best use of family, friends, and support networks so you don't face challenges alone.

- **Chapter 10: I Need to Keep Moving Forward**—bring it all together, adjust to new challenges, and move forward living with chronic illness.

A Little Pep Talk

Receiving a chronic illness diagnosis is a turning point. Yes, it is a profound change, and yes, it may feel as though you no longer belong in the "healthy" world. But you still belong in the world… the world of all individuals who are alive!

You are still you. You are still valuable. You are still part of life.

But what if you don't feel this way?

It's normal to feel scared, angry, or adrift at first. But this book is here to guide you toward acceptance, resilience, and—most importantly—hope.

Cut Yourself Some Slack Following Your Diagnosis

The period right after your diagnosis is often the hardest. The shock can be intense, and the urge to get back to "normal" may be just as strong. But cut yourself some slack and take your time. You know yourself best—whether you need to resume work and daily routines right away, or step back briefly to adjust, the choice is yours. Emotions may come in waves, sometimes unexpectedly, and that's natural. Allow yourself to experience them, whether by leaning on others for support or by taking quiet moments alone.

During this time, it's easy to feel overwhelmed or forget simple things. Writing reminders can help you stay grounded. Most importantly, remember that confusion and emotional ups and downs do settle over time. Awareness, understanding, and acceptance arrive gradually, at their own pace. You can ease this process — and strengthen your adjustment—by using the strategies outlined in this book to help you move forward with greater confidence.

How to Use This Book

This guide is not meant to be read cover to cover. Think of it as a toolbox. Skim the chapters to get a sense of the strategies available, then focus on the areas that matter most to you right now. You'll notice that there are brackets before each strategy number. As you skim through the book, check any of the strategies you want to use, as well as those that seem helpful and worthy of additional review.

Most strategies in this book include a "To Use This Strategy" section with specific steps suggested. For a smaller number, you won't see that section—their purpose is to offer perspective and encourage reflection (or discussion with your care team), giving you ideas that help you to keep moving forward and reclaim your life.

As new challenges arise in the future, you can return to the book, confident that additional strategies will be waiting for you when you need them.

Here are some suggestions for how to get the most out of this book:

- **Skim first, then dive in.** Familiarize yourself with the range of strategies before choosing where to begin. Check the ones you want to review further.
- **Pick what fits you.** Not every strategy will apply, but many can help you right away.
- **Adapt as needed.** Make each strategy your own; the best plan is the one that works for you.
- **Build over time.** Some strategies can be applied quickly, while others grow in benefit the more you practice them.
- **Seek support if needed.** Share this book with your healthcare team or a mental health professional to guide discussions and goals.

Remember: self-improvement requires action. Just saying you want to cope is not enough—you must do the work. This book is your action guide.

Are you ready? Let's begin the journey to living well after diagnosis.

I Need to Get Ready to Help Myself

Living with a chronic or serious illness can be a very difficult, life-altering experience. (This is an understatement!) Once you receive your diagnosis—or face new challenges with a condition you've been managing—the question becomes: how do you move forward? What should you do to regain a sense of control and cope more effectively?

As with any important project, the first step is preparation. The more prepared you are, the greater your chances of success. Preparation is the foundation for living well after diagnosis and for navigating your new reality with strength and resilience.

This chapter introduces some basic starting-point strategies. These are practical tools that can be used repeatedly, at any stage of your journey. They are designed to help you organize, reduce uncertainty, and strengthen your ability to cope. Think of these as the groundwork for you to cope, move forward, and begin reclaiming your life with chronic illness.

[ ] #1

Set Up Your Coping Notebook

One of the best ways for you to get started is to set up a Coping Notebook. Having everything in one place helps you feel more organized, reduces stress, and shows your healthcare team that you are an active partner in your care. There are a number of reasons for this:

First, it will keep all of the important information concerning your illness and your self-improvement efforts in one place.

Second, it will provide you with an ongoing resource to use for all of the strategies that you select and all of the results that you obtain.

Third, it will keep you focused on what you're trying to accomplish and will help you to monitor your progress as you achieve your goals.

And fourth, you'll have all of your information in one easy-to-carry resource to take to all of your appointments.

Not only will it help you to ask the questions you need to ask and write down the information you learn, it will also show any professional you're seeing that you truly are taking an active role in your life following your diagnosis.

Many of the strategies in this book include the suggestion to use your Coping Notebook. Set up your Coping Notebook as you choose. There is no right or wrong way. However, there are a few suggestions that can make this work best for you.

To use this strategy:

Use a loose-leaf notebook. In this way, you can add pages as necessary, and remove (or, at least, move to the back) pages that are no longer a priority.

Set up different sections. For example:

- A journal of your feelings and experiences
- A new page for each coping strategy you use
- A section for your healthcare professionals
- A section for your treatment components (medications, physical therapy, counseling, etc.)

These suggestions can make it easier for you to find important information without thumbing through every page.

When you find strategies that help you, keep using them as long as they're helpful… even after you finish your worksheet. Add blank sheets to your loose-leaf notebook to continue your work.

By the way, your Coping Notebook doesn't necessarily have to be in a paper format. You might prefer to set up a comprehensive document on your computer, tablet, or mobile device. This way, you can easily add or rearrange "pages," just as you would in a paper notebook. No matter the format, what matters most is that it functions as *your* Coping Notebook- a tool to help you stay organized, cope effectively, and regain a sense of control.

[ ] #2

Make Reminder Lists

There will be plenty of things to remember to do during the first days and weeks following your diagnosis. Not only can it be stressful to deal with your diagnosis, but it can also be overwhelming to worry that you're forgetting something. Writing things down reduces that risk, lightens your mental load, and gives you a real sense of accomplishment when you check items off.

To use this strategy:

Designate a place to keep your reminders. You can:

- Set up a section in your Coping Notebook.
- Keep a small notebook specifically for reminders.
- Use your smartphone or another device.
- Include details such as what the task is, when it needs to be done, how, and by whom. Each completed check mark reinforces control and forward progress… and can be very satisfying!

[ ] #3

Know When to Go into "Coping Mode"

After your diagnosis, you may feel like your life is spinning out of control.

So, what can you do to regain a sense of balance? What do you do when you feel you've hit a roadblock? The answer: go into "coping mode". This technique helps you separate overwhelming emotions from problem-solving action and empowers you to regain control in difficult moments.

By going into coping mode, you're telling yourself, "I am now going to figure out what I need to do to help myself, to better manage the situation."

To use this strategy:

Going into coping mode involves several simple steps:

- Identify the problem. What triggered your need to go into coping mode?
- Define your goal. What do you want to accomplish?

- Consider different options or strategies that may help you to accomplish your goal.
- Prioritize your options and decide what to try first. Writing down the steps or even creating a small contract with yourself, specifying what you're going to do, how, when, and other details, can be helpful.
- Work on the steps or options that you have selected for yourself.
- Review your results and make changes as needed
- Cross off the goals you complete (even if they are small steps) and reward yourself for progress. Use this as a motivator.

[ ] #4

Use the Double-Column Technique

The double-column technique is one of the most powerful and frequently used strategies to benefit you in your coping efforts. By laying out problems and solutions side by side, you train your brain to shift from negativity toward constructive action.

To use this strategy:

Fold a piece of paper (or use a page in your Coping Notebook) in half. On the left side, write down upsetting thoughts, goals, or questions. On the right side, write constructive responses, steps, or answers.

Here are a few examples of uses for the double-column technique.

- Upsetting thoughts vs. healthier ways of thinking. If you're having trouble with your thinking, you can write upsetting, negative thoughts on the left side of the page. On the right side, directly across from what you've written on the left side, write down more appropriate ways of thinking.
- Goals vs. steps needed to achieve them. If you've established a goal to work on, you can write that goal on the left side of the

page. On the right side of the page, write down the steps that you can use to achieve that goal.

- Questions for your doctor vs. answers you receive. If you have questions about your treatment, you can write them down on the left side of the page. Then, when you get the answers to your questions, you can write them down on the right side of the page.
- Relationships to improve vs. specific steps you might take. On the left side of the page, you can write down the names of people you want to improve relationships with. On the right side of the page, you can write down steps that you might take in order to accomplish that.

Throughout this book, there will be a number of strategies that suggest that you use the double-column technique. The way you use it is up to you, but you'll find it to be a very effective way to focus, organize, and improve your thinking.

[ ] #5

Learn About the Benefits of Using Relaxation Techniques

No matter how your diagnosis affects you, relaxation techniques can be a crucial, empowering first step. Relaxation techniques are important for several reasons:

- They can reduce or help you manage any stressors that may adversely affect or overwhelm you.
- They ease both the physical and emotional impact of stress.
- They can help to reduce some of the pain you may be experiencing.
- They can help you to immediately feel that you're DOING something to help yourself ... and it feels good!

There are many options:

- Progressive muscle relaxation: A 15- to 20-minute technique in which you sequentially tense and relax the different groups of muscles in your body, one group at a time.
- Meditation: A peaceful technique in which you focus your mind on a sound, word, object, or experience, while "clearing out" extraneous thoughts. Meditation not only reduces anxiety, it also keeps you focused in an empowering way.
- Guided imagery: The process of conjuring up mental images or scenes in order to help relax your body and mind. (See Strategy #7 for more information.)
- Yoga, tai chi, and similar body movement strategies: Techniques that involve breathing control, basic meditation, and physical postures, to alleviate stress and anxiety and improve health.
- Biofeedback: A technique that combines the strategies of relaxation and guided imagery with the use of electronic, "high-tech" measuring instruments.

There are plenty of ways to learn more—books, online programs, apps, or other resources. One relaxation technique that I developed more than 40 years ago, called the "Quick Release," is explained in more detail on the website page www.coping.com/quickrelease. Feel free to check out the instructions and try it.

[ ] #6

Begin Using Relaxation Techniques ... Regularly

Once you have decided which relaxation technique(s) you're going to start using, commit to the idea of using them regularly. The real benefit comes from consistency—training your body and mind to respond more effectively over time. You'll be amazed at how much better you'll feel.

You'll feel better physically (because learning how to relax can help to reduce the impact of virtually any physical symptom). And you'll feel better emotionally (because you'll realize that there are things you can do that can bring about immediate results, and you do still have some control over your life!).

Relaxation techniques can be used in two important ways: "preventatively" and "curatively." What does this mean?

As with all good skills, the more you use them, the more effective they are. By practicing your relaxation techniques, you get your body used to them and the way they work. It builds up your confidence in them, and you "condition" your body (you get your body used to the way relaxation feels) so it responds more quickly and effectively to future uses of the technique. This can help you preventatively. In other words, this can prevent or decrease the likelihood of stress, anxiety, or other symptoms, because you've practiced and are prepared.

However, what if something does happen, or you experience stress or another symptom? That is when you can use your relaxation technique curatively. This refers to using your relaxation technique to try to regain control at the first sign of a problem. It's your attempt to improve your ability to deal with a currently occurring situation or symptom.

To use this strategy:

Write your plan in your Coping Notebook. Schedule daily relaxation activities, such as progressive muscle relaxation before bed or guided imagery during a lunch break. If you're going to use a technique more than once a day (which is especially helpful early on), schedule those times in advance. In your Coping Notebook, write down how you felt, what worked, and what you'd like to adjust. The more you practice, the more you'll benefit.

[ ] #7

Use Guided Imagery

Guided imagery (also called visualization) involves creating a detailed, vivid image in your mind. It taps into the mind-body connection, easing symptoms, reducing pain, and giving you a coping tool you can control anytime and anywhere.

Research has shown that there is a very strong connection between the body and the mind. The more vividly you visualize something, the more likely it is that you may get some physical benefit from this strategy. For example, guided imagery has been proven to be helpful in reducing physical pain.

To use this strategy:

Set aside a few quiet minutes and give yourself permission to experiment—there's no single "right" image. Any images, sensations, or even words that are meaningful to you can work. The simple steps below will guide you. Notice what helps, jot it down in your Coping Notebook, and repeat regularly to build the skill.

- Identify your goal. Are you trying to imagine a general feeling of physical comfort? Are you trying to work on a particular symptom? Are you just trying to relax? There are as many goals for guided imagery as there are people using it.
- Practice guided imagery in a quiet, distraction-free environment. (Obviously, distractions are not relaxing and can interfere with what you're trying to accomplish.) Guided imagery tends to work better with your eyes closed, so you can block out anything else that you might see that could interfere with your planned visual images.

- Use deep, rhythmic, relaxed breathing. Not only does this feel good, but it will get your mind more receptive to the guided imagery you're going to create.
- "Paint a picture." Make your guided imagery as vivid and as real as you can. But remember, this is guided imagery, so you can create whatever mental images you feel would be helpful. (They don't have to be anatomically or physiologically correct!)
- Immerse yourself in your created image(s). In addition to visualizing it, incorporate all of your senses (hearing, smell, touch, etc.) in your image.
- If you're using guided imagery for a particular symptom, create images to gently and gradually reverse the symptom. You can even conclude your guided imagery by visualizing something exceptionally soothing.
- Practice your guided imagery regularly. Repetition leads to progress.

Here are a few examples: If you're experiencing pain, you might imagine a healing warmth surrounding the affected area and gradually soothing it. If you're anxious, you might picture yourself at a calm beach, hearing the waves, feeling the sun, and breathing slowly. The more detail you use, the more effective the exercise becomes.

Some people are able to use guided imagery better than others. Don't be discouraged if, at first, you're not "seeing" what you want to see. This is a skill, after all, that may need to be developed. It can take time to do better. Consider working with an expert on this technique if you feel guided imagery could be beneficial, but you're having a hard time using it.

[ ] #8

Learn How to Effectively Distract Yourself

There may be times when you're upset about something that's happening, or the way you're thinking, and there's nothing that you can do about the situation. It's at those times that you would be best served by being able to briefly distract yourself from any of the negative thoughts or feelings that arise because of the situation you're in. Distraction interrupts negative thoughts, creating space for more positive thinking and emotional recovery.

To use this strategy:

There are a variety of ways you can distract yourself. You can get involved with an activity (doing a chore, making a phone call, writing an e-mail), use guided imagery (picture yourself someplace relaxing, or having fun with friends), or focus on something specific and neutral (look at the color and texture of the chair you're sitting in. Really look at it.).

There are other examples of more prolonged distraction techniques, including listening to music, watching a favorite TV show, working on a hobby, or calling a supportive friend. For any of them, the key is to give your mind a different focus long enough to interrupt the cycle of negative thoughts.

[ ] #9

Use the Channel-Changing Strategy

What can you do if you keep thinking about something and you want to move away from that type of thinking? Consider using something I call the "channel-changing" strategy. This can be used for distraction, but it can also be used as a focusing strategy. Imagining a mental "channel change" allows you to consciously redirect your focus toward healthier, calmer, or more empowering thoughts.

To use this strategy:

Imagine that the situation you're in (including what you're doing, thinking, or reacting to) is on one channel. If that channel is uncomfortable for you, or you recognize the need to change the way you're thinking or what you're doing, consciously make the decision to change the channel. Change it to something that's peaceful, relaxing, or empowering.

For example, if your "channel" is filled with worries about an upcoming medical test, you might mentally "switch" to a channel where you're remembering a family gathering or imagining a future goal you're excited about. Just like changing the TV channel with a remote, you're reminding yourself that you have choices in what you focus on.

This technique works best if you plan in advance what your "coping channel" is going to be. You may want to visualize doing this in your mind, and practice it, so you're more familiar and prepared with what you're going to do at those times when you need to cope by changing channels.

WHAT'S NEXT?

Living with a chronic illness can feel overwhelming—physically, emotionally, and practically. It may seem impossible to take it all in at once. That's okay. Start small, remind yourself that every step matters, and know that each bit of progress builds a stronger foundation. The next chapter will help you understand your reactions to your diagnosis and begin absorbing the knowledge you need to move forward.

CHAPTER 2

I Need to Understand What's Happening

Now that you've read about some of the basic strategies to get started, the next step in living well after diagnosis is to try to grasp what's going on. This may sound very simplistic, but it makes sense. You want to understand what is happening to your body, and you want to understand what this illness is all about.

Your diagnosis may have knocked you for a loop. That's normal. But knowledge is power. Understanding provides clarity, reduces fear, and gives you a stronger foundation for moving forward. This chapter will guide you through strategies to process your initial and subsequent reactions, and to educate yourself so that you feel informed, empowered, and better prepared to cope with your illness.

A- Initial Reactions

There are many different reactions that you may experience at the time of diagnosis. For example:

- You may feel terrified, worrying about what's going to happen next, as well as in the future.
- You may feel isolated, as if you're now on the "outside looking in."

- You may cry, or you may get angry.
- You may want to go to sleep.
- You may call your friends, contact family members, or play with the dog.
- You may feel a variety of other emotions, including loneliness, sadness, confusion, or even hopelessness.

Any of these reactions are perfectly normal.

You may even feel relief. Why? It may have taken you a long time to be diagnosed. There may have been many other things that you feared while you were waiting for your diagnosis. So, you might feel relieved that now, at least, there's a label attached to your symptoms. Now you can get treated and try to proceed in a positive direction.

So, what do you need to understand first? Let's start with the strategies.

[ ] #10

Ride Out the Shock of Your Diagnosis

Most people feel shocked when they're first diagnosed with a chronic illness. Even though you may have suspected it, having a name attached to it can be shocking. Acknowledging this shock as normal reduces self-blame and reassures you that adjustment will come with time.

Your goal should be to get past the shock (and you will!) and learn how to deal with all the manifestations of the diagnosis.

Your first question may naturally be, "Why this diagnosis? Why, why, why???" Wanting to know why is a common first reaction. (And, of course, the inevitable "why me?" questions, which will be addressed in Strategy #31.)

When you initially ask yourself, "Where did this illness come from?" there may be a variety of possible answers. They might include family history, environmental causes, an accident, a related condition, or a variety of other possibilities. Or there may be no explanations as to why this occurred.

It's possible that you're not even expecting a specific answer. Rather, you're releasing frustration that something like this has blindsided you.

You may experience shock at other times during the course of your disease, though usually to a lesser extent, if you experience any major changes or reversals. If that happens, you'll want to use the appropriate coping strategies then as well.

[ ] #11
Face Your Diagnosis Head On

The best way to start moving in the right direction is to face the fact that you now have this illness. You've been diagnosed. You've got this condition. Facing reality directly helps you move past denial, so you can begin focusing on constructive action.

It is normal to hope and pray that your doctors have made a mistake. You may intellectually know that you've been diagnosed with a chronic illness. But you may not emotionally "get" it. This is what keeps your initial progress slow.

The best advice is to stay focused on what you intellectually know, even if you're having a hard time dealing with it emotionally.

Having a better understanding of where the disease came from can help you cope with the diagnosis. Then, you can start focusing on your specific symptoms and, more importantly, your treatment.

The initial shock of being diagnosed will gradually go away as you adjust to the reality of having the disease.

[ ] #12

Write Down the Way You Feel

This is one of the key initial strategies. When you are hit with the diagnosis of a medical problem, the shock can be overwhelming. Try to put your feelings into words. Journaling provides a catharsis or emotional release, increases self-awareness, and helps track your progress over time. This can be very beneficial.

Some people are afraid to write these things down because it makes the diagnosis "real". They believe this "confirms" the diagnosis, and they're still hoping that it isn't true. However, by writing your feelings down, you are taking an important step in admitting that you have this (and that is something you need to do).

To use this strategy:

Set up a page in your Coping Notebook entitled, "How Am I Feeling?" Date it and then begin, just letting your thoughts flow onto paper. Don't try to editorialize or proofread as you go, and don't worry about anyone else reading it (unless you want them to.)

Then, when you have finished writing down your thoughts, ask yourself what do you want to do with this? Some people use it as a springboard to positive action. Some people don't want to look at it ever again. Some people use it as the basis to ask questions of their doctors. Some people keep it in their Coping Notebook so they can refer to it and see how they've made progress. You will figure out the best uses for you.

You may choose to use this strategy over and over, whenever something else occurs that triggers an onslaught of thoughts and emotions.

[ ] #13

Anticipate a Variety of Emotional Reactions

A diagnosis can create a myriad of emotional reactions. You may feel like your head is spinning. Knowing that emotions will fluctuate prevents surprise and helps you prepare healthy responses in advance.

Following your diagnosis, your emotions will be all over the place. As you learn more about your disease, how to take care of yourself, go through some of the symptomatic manifestations of the disease, and experience treatment, you'll experience an unpredictable variety of emotions.

For example, your anger will fluctuate. Even if you're extremely angry about having a chronic illness, this intense anger will not last forever (even if your condition does). There will be times when you're feeling angrier, but other times you may feel calmer and more matter-of-fact about what you're going through. Of course, during these more matter-of-fact times, you may hope you'll never feel that anger again. Don't bank on that. There may be times when anger returns, for many different reasons.

There are other emotions that you may feel because of the diagnosis, including:

- You may feel depressed, feeling that your life will never be the same.
- You may feel anxious about symptoms, treatment, the future, or more.
- You may feel sadness because you feel so overwhelmed with the changes that are a necessity.
- You may feel stress or confusion because of these changes, and how much you're going to need to know and do to take care of yourself.

- You may feel guilty about being more of a burden on your family.
- You may experience other feelings, such as being lost, helpless, hopeless, or overwhelmed.

The way you see yourself (your self-esteem) and your body (your body image) may change. How and why does this happen?

- You may feel stigmatized because you have an illness.
- You may feel that you're not the same person as you were.
- You may feel that you don't look the same to others or yourself.
- You may feel that others look at you differently.
- You may feel like you are not a whole person anymore.
- You might be embarrassed or ashamed that you've been diagnosed with this illness.

You may go through a variety of other reactions and emotions as you adjust to your diagnosis. These are all normal reactions, and, fortunately, are usually short-lived. Knowing this should help you to be less surprised if you have any of these reactions. You'll then be in a better position to do something to help yourself to deal with them.

Believe it or not, it's up to you how you allow these feelings to affect you and remain with you. The strategies in this book will help you to deal with them.

Indeed, your disease is not something you want. However, it is now a part of your life. Know that, with time, you will be better able to cope with the fact that your illness is now a part of you.

Initially, it may feel like your chronic illness is controlling you. But fortunately, you will find that the more you learn and can do for yourself, the more normal and in control you will feel. You will grow to accept your illness as being part of you, even if you don't like it.

[ ] #14

Start Dealing with Any Emotional Distress

Rarely does somebody experience the diagnosis of a chronic illness without it affecting them emotionally. However, the degree to which this affects you may also depend on how you were handling your emotions before the diagnosis.

If you were affected by emotional turmoil before your diagnosis, you may find that you have a harder time dealing with your diagnosis. If your self-esteem is low, you might say something like, "What else is going to happen to me?" Even if you were relatively stress-free and were dealing well with your life as it was, the diagnosis of a chronic illness can still be devastating.

So, what else can be distressing? To somebody who was seemingly relatively healthy five minutes ago, the diagnosis may make you worry about a bad outcome. You may worry about being the person who has all the complications, and your life will never be the same. Everybody has their own emotional reactions to their own diagnosis.

The emotions that you experience following the diagnosis can change from day to day, even moment to moment. Up-and-down cycles are very common. The goal is to try to smooth out your path as you come to grips with your chronic illness. One of the best ways to start doing this is by changing your negative thoughts to more realistic, positive ones, using a rewriting technique called cognitive restructuring.

To use this strategy:

On a page in your Coping Notebook, use the double-column technique (Strategy #4) to write down and describe any emotion you're feeling. Then, ask yourself what you're thinking that is making you feel that way. These negative thoughts should be written on the left side of the page. Leave a few lines between each negative thought. Then, on the right side of the page, write down a better way of thinking in response.

If you're unable to come up with a response, ask yourself what someone you respect would say to comfort you. Or, what would you say to a friend in your shoes? Keep referring to your responses on this page when you find yourself overwhelmed emotionally. Continue using this strategy and not only will your thinking improve, but your emotions will as well.

If you still have trouble responding to your emotion-inducing thoughts, you may find it helpful to talk to a mental health professional who can help you learn better and healthier ways of thinking.

[ ] #15

Recognize How "Protective Barriers" Help Deal with Information Overload

It is not unusual, in the days following a diagnosis, to feel overwhelmed by everything you're hearing. The diagnosis itself, treatment strategies, everything that you have to do, and more, can come together in a way that makes you feel inundated with scary information.

The mind often reacts to this stressful feeling by erecting an emotional "barrier" to protect itself from "too much input." That may sound fine, except that if you experience this, you may feel detached from your "normal" world or feel "on the outside looking in". You may worry that you're losing it, or even that you're having a breakdown.

So, what should you do? Remind yourself that this is an unfortunate feeling, but it's part of the process of absorbing the enormity of your diagnosis and understanding all of the facts that you need to know. It may take a little time, but you will get to a point where your emotional barrier is less and less necessary.

Discuss any difficulties with your doctor. If you're really feeling overwhelmed, there are professionals who may be able to provide you with support and know-how. You may also want to discuss the possibility of taking medication to help you cope with it.

Reassure yourself that, despite it feeling very unpleasant, this protective barrier is normal ... and temporary. This feeling will pass. Recognizing that this often is an instinctive response to information overload will help you to get through it.

[ ] #16
Grieve Your Loss

When people are diagnosed with a chronic condition, they do experience a loss: the loss of their health the way it was before the diagnosis. This feels as real for them as grieving the loss of a loved one. Anticipate that. You will go through stages of grieving similar to what people go through when they lose a loved one. Grieving acknowledges the reality of your loss and allows you to move toward acceptance and healing.

Here are the five commonly referred to stages of grieving:

- Shock and denial (trying to believe that mistakes have been made, that this isn't happening to you)
- Anger (the "Why me?" stage)
- Bargaining (for example, "If I'm a better person, or I eat healthier, my diagnosis will change.")
- Depression (This can occur as one starts to face the reality that the diagnosis is real.)
- Acceptance (the ultimate goal-- not liking, but accepting, the diagnosis, and knowing this is part of you)

These stages are normal. Every person diagnosed with a chronic illness goes through them. However, each person goes through them differently and may spend different lengths of time in each stage. Some may go back to previous stages or, seemingly, skip a stage.

Each person is different. There's no one formula for how people progress through the stages. There is no timetable to follow. So, don't have expectations of how you're going to go through the five stages, or how long it's going to take. Rather, just try to understand that it's a process. You'll go through it…and get through it.

You can help yourself with this process. What's the common denominator in all of these stages? The way you think. So, if you find yourself trying to figure out how to get to the acceptance stage, start by working to improve your thinking. We'll discuss much more about this in a number of strategies in this book. In addition, this is an area in which speaking to a counselor can be very helpful.

[ ] #17

Learn How to Let Go in Order to Move Forward

One of the biggest difficulties following the diagnosis of chronic illness is the feeling that your life has changed. No matter how you felt about your life before, you may be even more upset and apprehensive about what's to come.

Letting go of unrealistic expectations frees you to build a meaningful, joyful life, even though you have a chronic illness.

Yes, your life will be different, but that doesn't mean it can't be great. Yes, you'll encounter obstacles. (Everybody does.) It's important to let go…not of your dreams, but of any expectations you have had that your life would be uneventful, stable, and with no obstacles. Instead, embrace the idea of change, encouraging yourself to believe that, yes, it may be different, but it can be better!

You may be thinking, "How can my life be better?" It can if you want it to. There are people who take adversities in life and turn them into something positive. They use it to motivate them to go on to do things they have always wanted to do but never got around to doing. Wouldn't you want to be that person?

Write the book you always wanted to write, work on having a better relationship with a loved one, learn something new, smell the roses, etc. Do whatever it is that you can, within your limitations, to make your life better and happier. Control your destiny instead of letting it control you.

Here's one of my favorite mottos (yes, you can quote me!):"You have to let go of what was, and what could have been… in order to enjoy what is, and what still can be!" Make this the cornerstone of your efforts to adjust to your diagnosis. Repeat it to yourself, over and over.

B- Learn About Your Illness

So, how much do you know about your illness? Immediately following your diagnosis, you may feel that you know very little (or practically nothing) about your condition. You may only know what you heard about it from a family member, a friend with this condition, or in the news.

Doesn't it make sense to learn as much as you can about your condition? After all, what you experience may be different from what others experience.

Once you are diagnosed, you may be overwhelmed by how much information exists about your condition, how much you need to learn, and how scary all of this may be. Start slowly. Ask your doctor to tell you the most important things about your condition that you should take away from your appointment. That will give you a good place to start.

The strategies in this section will help you to become more knowledgeable about your illness…a very important part of coping.

[ ] #18

Do a "Symptom Inventory"

There are many ways in which your newly diagnosed condition may affect your body. Since each person and each condition is different, each person may experience different symptoms.

Part of dealing with your illness is learning what you can about your symptoms. To start doing this, it can be helpful to do a "Symptom Inventory." You'll keep track of details about your symptoms, and you'll then be able to use this information to discuss treatment strategies with your medical team.

Tracking symptoms equips you to give your healthcare team clear information and improves treatment planning.

To use this strategy:

In your Coping Notebook, make a list of each symptom you're currently experiencing. Include as much information as you can. For example, indicate the "FID" about each symptom (the frequency, intensity, and duration), as well as how important it is to you to attend to this symptom.

Then, indicate any responses you get from your treatment team about each symptom. Keep records of what treatment modalities or medications are being used to address each symptom, as well as the results.

[ ] #19

Keep a Question Log

As you go through the days and weeks following your diagnosis, questions will inevitably pop into your head. These questions may arise because of things you're experiencing, things you hear or read, comments from others, or anticipating medical appointments. These questions may have to do with virtually any facet of your life that is affected by the diagnosis.

Writing down questions ensures you remember them, get clearer answers, and stay engaged as your own advocate.

Anything can cause a question to pop into your mind. Whatever the cause, keep a list of these questions. If it's significant, you may even want to note what caused the question to occur to you.

No one knows all of the questions they need to ask. The more informed you become about your illness, the more questions you'll likely have. You'll become more aware of them as time goes by, following your diagnosis.

Don't expect that you're going to have your questions answered all at once. That's why it is so helpful to write them down as they occur, so you can return to them later as new information becomes available.

To use this strategy:

Set up a question/answer page to keep track of your questions... and the answers that you obtain. This will help you to develop your own "resource guide" of questions and answers.

Examples of initial questions you'll likely want answers to include:

- What is the name of your condition?
- How does it affect your body?
- What causes your condition?
- How does the condition typically progress?
- What causes this condition to progress or get worse?
- What tests and procedures are typically used to determine the course of your treatment?
- What treatments are available for your condition?
- What are the treatments actually supposed to do?
- What is involved in your prescribed treatment?
- What complications and side effects might occur with each treatment?
- What are some of the more unusual complications and side effects that you'd need to report to your doctor?
- How will this impact your usual day-to-day activities?
- And, of course, the question you may be most afraid to ask: What is the prognosis?

Know who you're going to ask these questions, so that you can get the best possible answers for them. By writing them down, you are one step closer to the answers. It will help to keep you focused on what you want to ask your physician during your next office visit, or by telephone. You may want to take someone with you to your next office visit so that they can remind you to ask these questions. In addition, it's a good idea to have someone else with you to hear the answers in case you forget what they were, and also to give you a different perspective on the answers. (See Strategy #106.)

By keeping track of your questions, it will also help you to determine resources other than your physician (such as a pharmacist, or other health professional), or even non-medical people (such as an attorney, accountant, or support group leader) who you may want (or need) to ask questions.

To review: make sure you write down the answers you receive. Because you're still early in your learning process, and you still may be emotionally overwhelmed, you may not absorb or remember everything you hear. Also, when you review the answers, more questions may be triggered. Write them down as well.

[ ] #20

Become an Expert About Your Condition

Although your initial goal may not have been for you to know everything there is to know about your condition, you'll find that the more you know, the more empowered you will be to help yourself get back on your feet.

Knowledge empowers you to make better choices, ask informed questions, and feel more in control.

The preliminary information that you find out, including answers to the questions you've asked, is important as a foundation for living following your diagnosis.

You don't have to obtain this information all at once, and you don't always have to do extensive research into medical literature to get the answers. You can ask your doctors and other experts and obtain information using other resources suggested in subsequent strategies (such as Strategy #23.)

Once you have general information about your condition, based on your research and consultation with others, you'll then want to start finding out how that information applies in your situation.

Use your Coping Notebook to keep track of all the details you learn about your condition. Your goal is to learn as much as you possibly can about your disease. Even when you think you know everything there is to know, remember this: You don't! Keep on learning.

Don't expect to ever know everything about your condition. No one does (not even the doctors!). Yes, a reasonable goal is to know as much as you can, so you are in the best position to help yourself. You want to be your own best advocate. But be realistic about how much you can expect to learn, especially at the outset.

To use this strategy:

Make two lists. The first is a list of the things that you currently know about your condition. (This may seem foolish, but you'll realize how important it is as you get into the strategy.)

The second list is of the things that you don't know or need to know. Indicate how you're going to find answers to these items or questions that you may have.

Keep an ongoing list of questions that may occur to you. Answer as many of them as you can, when you can. There are times when there may not be specific or obtainable answers. But then these questions remain open for additional research or consultation.

Include a list of questions that you want to ask your doctor. The more specific the questions, the better. But your doctor is not the only resource you can use to accumulate information. (See Strategy #23 for suggestions.)

This will be an ongoing process. The list may change depending on any changes in your condition, your symptoms, or your treatment. As you learn things from the second list, you can move those items to the first list.

[ ] #21

Determine When You're Ready to Learn More

It might make sense that as soon as you're diagnosed, you immediately try to get as much information as you can. But emotionally, you may not be ready. So, it really depends on you. You may need to learn as you're ready to learn. As long as you don't put this off too long, you can start the process of learning about your condition when the time is right for you.

What if you find that questions pop into your head, even though you're not prepared to find out the answers? Write down the questions anyway. Use the question-and-answer strategy. (See Strategy #19.) This will help you to know that at least you're taking some steps, even if you're not ready to obtain information to answer your questions.

[ ] #22

Take What You Hear About Your Illness with a "Grain of Salt"

As you obtain information about your condition, you may hear things that are unpleasant or uncomfortable for you to hear. Some of this may be important for you to know, but some of it may just not be necessary for you, especially right now. So, take what you hear (and read) with a grain of salt.

This is yet another reason why it's very important to use appropriate resources for content, as well as to filter information from well-meaning individuals.

Use your intelligence and good judgment to figure out if what you're reading or hearing makes sense, is pertinent, and best meets your needs.

To use this strategy:

Use your double-column technique for this. For example, if you hear something and you're not sure if it is accurate or relevant for you, write it on the left side of the page. Then on the right side of the page, write down your reaction to it. For example, is this something you want to pursue, to learn more about, to ask your doctor, or is it something for you to dismiss?

You're going to be bombarded with plenty of information and opinions, especially immediately following your diagnosis. You should figure out a way to distinguish between valuable information and information that is dismissible.

[ ] #23

Use Reliable Resources

So, where do you go, and what do you do to learn about your condition? Information about your condition, or treatment for your condition, can be obtained from a variety of resources. In all cases, make sure all of the information you obtain is current and reliable. Resources include:

- Your healthcare professionals
- Health-related organizations and agencies
- Other organizations (depending on your needs)
- Hospitals or research centers
- Books. (Books also contain references, resources, and appendices that may provide additional information or leads.)
- Newspapers (especially suggestions for agencies or self-help groups that might be beneficial)
- People, including social networks, support groups, and others who have or are dealing with your disease
- And, of course, the internet. (See Strategy #24.)

To use this strategy:

Be a detective. There is so much information out there; you should continue to pursue different options. Be selective, prioritize, and don't overwhelm yourself.

Even if you obtain valuable information from one source, it's good to balance it with information that you get from other sources. Ask anyone whose opinion you respect what resources you should consult to start learning more about your condition. Network with other people you know. Remember, you're not the first person to ask these questions. Don't hesitate to ask the questions you need answered.

As you obtain information, make sure to keep it in one place. That will make it easier to refer to any time you have any questions or need to look something up. It's a good idea to write the most important information in your Coping Notebook.

[ ] #24
Learn from Trusted Websites

The internet can be a very valuable resource. (After all, you're able to accumulate so much information from the comfort of your chair... or bed!) But you need to use it wisely.

Trusted websites from hospitals, universities, and government health agencies provide accurate, up-to-date information you can rely on. Using these sources helps you stay informed without being misled by rumors, outdated advice, or frightening worst-case scenarios.

To use this strategy:

Initially, spend some time determining which reputable online sites you're going to browse. Ask people you're working with (e.g., doctors or nurses), or people who deal with your condition (e.g., in health organizations or support groups) for suggestions for good websites to visit.

Check out information that comes from large hospital systems, such as the Mayo Clinic, the Cleveland Clinic, Johns Hopkins, among others.

Look for information from other large institutions that are currently active in dealing with your disease.

Look for "refereed" journals (meaning that any articles are professionally reviewed and approved by experts before they're even published). A well-known example of a refereed journal is the New England Journal of Medicine. Many such journals are available on the internet.

Other resources include government-produced information, such as from the NIH (National Institutes of Health) or the CDC (Center for Disease Control and Prevention).

In your Coping Notebook, create a page for internet-based resources. List the sites you trust and note the key points you find there. This way, you'll know where to return for reliable information, instead of endlessly scrolling.

[ ] #25

Use Trusted Digital Tools

The internet is full of information about every illness under the sun. Some of it is helpful, but much of it is unreliable or even harmful. A late-night search can send you spiraling into worry over the worst-case scenarios, many of which don't even apply to your situation. It's natural to want answers, but it's just as important to make sure those answers come from trustworthy places.

Trusted digital tools — such as reputable websites, symptom-tracking apps, or medication reminders, or many others — can give you reliable knowledge and peace of mind while helping you stay organized. Used wisely, these resources expand your understanding, support your self-care, and prevent the confusion and discouragement that comes from misinformation.

To use this strategy:

Build a small, dependable toolkit you can turn to when questions pop up. The quick steps below will help you choose credible sources, keep them handy, and know what to do if something you read online raises concerns.

- Ask your doctor, nurse, or pharmacist which websites and apps they recommend.
- Pick just a few reliable sources—maybe two or three—and stick with them instead of scrolling endlessly.
- Bookmark your sources (or save them to Favorites) for quick access when questions arise.
- If something online worries you, write it down in your Coping Notebook and bring it to your next appointment rather than trying to interpret it alone.

[ ] #26
Be Wary of Promises of a Cure

In the previous two strategies, we discussed the value of the internet in obtaining information. But remember, some websites offer advice that is more accurate and reliable than others. Some diseases have dozens and dozens of websites devoted to "cures," and you may run a major risk of getting incorrect, possibly damaging, information that may not even apply to you.

Remember the old saying, "If it sounds too good to be true, it usually is." Avoid reading, or especially relying on, poorly written or unsolicited advice. There is a lot of hearsay and misguided advice out there that is not backed by scientific expertise.

When you're looking for information, rely on dependable, evidence-based sources—major hospitals, government health agencies, or respected disease-specific organizations—rather than first-person stories that push a "miracle cure." Strong emotions can make anyone more vulnerable to big promises; being aware of that helps you stay grounded.

Be especially cautious with claims that guarantee results, urge you to buy now, or tell you to stop prescribed treatments. If a cure were proven and relevant to your condition, your healthcare team would discuss it with you, and reputable medical sources would report it. In short: protect yourself from misinformation so your energy goes to what truly helps.

To use this strategy:

When you see a claim about a "new cure," pause and evaluate it before reacting. Check who published it (major hospital, government health agency, or disease-specific nonprofit vs. a personal blog or sales page), whether it's recent, and whether it cites real studies.

Be wary of red flags—testimonials instead of evidence, dramatic promises ("miracle," "breakthrough"), pressure to buy now, or advice to stop prescribed treatment.

In your Coping Notebook, jot the link, what it promises, and your questions. Don't start or stop any treatment (including supplements) based on what you read. Instead, bring the item to your next medical appointment—or send a portal message—and ask your doctor, nurse, or pharmacist, "Does this apply to me?"

Stick to a small set of trusted sites you've bookmarked. If a claim isn't confirmed there, treat it as unproven and move on.

[ ] #27

Act with the Best Information at Hand

As we've discussed, no one knows everything about your condition. At some point, you will need to act on the best information currently available. This would include recommendations and suggestions from those professionals whom you trust.

While you don't want to put energy into second-guessing yourself or replaying everything in hindsight, there are times when you need to "jump into the pool"—and begin taking action based on what you know now. You can always learn more as the days and weeks go by, and modify your approach accordingly.

Obviously, as you attempt to gain as much knowledge as you can about your condition, try not to be one of those people who delay making decisions about treatment (or even lifestyle changes) excessively, under the guise of waiting until they obtain still more information. In some cases, this may be absolutely a valid thing to do. In other cases, the "need" for additional information may be more of a delay tactic, in an attempt to avoid making decisions. This may contribute to a delay in obtaining necessary treatment.

Be honest with yourself. You know if you're trying to delay decision-making. If you are, try to figure out why you might be doing that. What are your concerns? What's holding you back?

This should probably be discussed honestly with your doctor. You may need to set goals and timetables for yourself so that you don't delay your decision-making too long.

C- Subsequent Reactions

After the initial shock resulting from your diagnosis, you may ask, "Now what?" You've begun the process of learning about your newly diagnosed condition. But this may lead to a new range of emotional reactions. These too may feel very intense, uncontrollable, and eternal. This is normal.

As time goes by, you'll be better able to deal with all of this realistically and positively. For right now, in order to get to that point, there are strategies to better deal with these subsequent reactions.

[ ] #28

Anticipate the Ups and Downs

Coming to grips with your diagnosis is like being on a roller coaster. You go through twists and turns, and ups and downs, and you can never fully anticipate what will occur, or when. There are times when you'll be able to cope, and others when you may feel you can't.

Remember that this roller coaster is normal. Practically everyone diagnosed with a chronic illness goes through it. Be prepared and develop strategies for how you will deal with this.

Eventually, the ride will get easier and smoother, and you will be better able to handle your diagnosis. All you have to do is look around at the people who have been able to deal with their conditions and remind yourself that you will be able to do so too. Following the strategies in this book will facilitate this process.

You will find that the emotional intensity of your diagnosis will fade over time. There may be times when it increases (possibly due to changes in symptom intensity, the need for new medical treatment, or other triggers). As you learn how to use your strategies to better cope with your diagnosis, you will be better able to smooth out this emotional swing.

There are many strategies in this book that will help you get through these ups and downs. You'll learn what's best for you, what helps when you're up, and what supports you when you're down. Being prepared will help you get through this more comfortably.

[ ] #29

Deal with The Out-of-Control Feelings

No matter how well you're dealing with things, there may be times when you feel overwhelmed or out of control. For example, there could be a "perfect storm" of symptoms and manifestations that overpower you. Reassure yourself that no matter how difficult these episodes may be, you can get through them. Stay focused and find something positive to concentrate on.

To use this strategy:

Should you find yourself getting one of these feelings, try to identify one positive thing that you can focus on. It might be someone in your family or a special event. It might be a hobby that you enjoy. It might be recalling a favorite scene in a movie or a passage in a book. Choose whatever feels grounding in that moment.

As these thoughts come to mind, write them down in your Coping Notebook, because they can be of help to you at future times if your feelings seem to be all over the place.

If you encounter a time when it is really difficult to think straight, the smart move is to reach out to significant others for their support.

Indicate in your Coping Notebook who you'd reach out to if you feel this way. In addition, mental health professionals can help you stay focused and manage those feelings. Keep contact information for any of these individuals easily accessible.

[ ] #30

Be Prepared for an Out-of-the-Blue Reaction

There may be times, as you're learning how to cope with your diagnosis, that you feel that you're starting to get a handle on it. Then, out of the blue, comes an intense, emotional reaction, possibly even without an identifiable trigger. This may scare you. Not only might it be a strong reaction, but it may also cast doubt on the progress you thought you had made in dealing with all of this.

Think positively. Recognize that any of these unexpected reactions are temporary. Yes, they may come, but they will also go.

To use this strategy:

In your Coping Notebook, jot down notes about any of these reactions that you experience. Include any relevant circumstances that you can identify. (If you have no idea what triggered it, include this as well.) Then, jot down ideas about what you can do to bounce back from this type of response. Not only will this help you with the current reaction, it will also help you deal with any future similar responses.

[ ] #31

Prepare Yourself for "Why Me" Questions

"Why me?" is probably the most common question people diagnosed with a chronic illness ask (more often to themselves than to others). Yet there is no simple answer, other than, "Why not me?"

Although these questions and comments are very common, think about how impractical they are. Are you truly going to come up with answers? No. Is it productive to think this way? No. That doesn't mean that you won't have these questions. But putting energy into trying to figure out answers that don't exist is counterproductive.

Think about it another way: Throughout your life, when good things happen, do you ask yourself, "Why me?" Of course not. Instead, you just enjoy those good things.

So, put your energy into figuring out how to best handle your current situation. Be constructive and proactive. Focus on the fact that it is what it is, and your job is to make the best of it.

[ ] #32

Anticipate Confusion and Unpredictability

There may be many different things about a diagnosis of a chronic illness that can be frustrating and confusing. Expect this. Take whatever steps you can to gather as much information as you reasonably can to reduce confusion.

Also, there are things that will arise as you live with your newly diagnosed condition that you can't anticipate, things that are unpredictable. Keep yourself flexible and ready to confront and conquer any of these changes. This will help you to get through them more effectively. Your goal? To be able to adjust as best you can. Roll with the punches.

[ ] #33

Be Mindful When Your Mind Is Wandering

Your goal in being mindful is to focus your full attention on what is going on in the present moment. At the same time, be aware and accepting of your feelings, thoughts, and physical sensations.

Why is this so important? When you start thinking too far down the road, contemplating all the things you need to cope with, all the things that could go wrong, as well as everything you have to do, it's easy to understand how overwhelmed you can be.

To use this strategy:

Stay focused on the present. Pay attention to what is happening now and what requires your attention. You're not ignoring the future; you're just saying that you will tackle it as it arrives, and in the meantime, you're facing the present moment.

Being mindful also implies accepting that "it is what it is", a very important goal for anyone dealing with the diagnosis of a chronic illness. This keeps you from being judgmental or dwelling on the "rightness or wrongness" of what's going on, or how you feel. Rather, it helps you to focus on what you're doing right now.

The goal is to consciously and deliberately focus on the "here and now," instead of reliving the past or worrying about the future.

D- Helping Your Understanding

So far in this chapter, you've learned how to deal with first reactions and the basics of initially understanding your condition. This section includes additional strategies to help you improve your ability to understand and deal with your diagnosis.

[ ] #34

Prepare for Challenges Ahead

It's hard enough to get a handle on all of the shock and emotions that come after the diagnosis of a chronic illness. Although everyone would like things to go smoothly after finally getting over the initial shock of the diagnosis, it rarely works that way. However, you can get through this, and you can help yourself by being prepared.

There are challenges that will occur along the path to successful living with your chronic illness. It's inevitable. By knowing this, and being ready to implement your coping strategies, you'll be able to better deal with these challenges.

What are some of the difficulties you may experience? There can be physical issues, new symptoms or treatment, lifestyle changes, social changes, family problems, financial issues, and emotional ups and downs, among others. (You'll find strategies to help you deal with many of these specific issues elsewhere in the book.)

Although there can be many different types of problems, don't expect to have to face all of them! Understand that challenges will occur, and the more you're prepared, the better you will be able to deal with them.

[ ] #35
Be Your Own Advocate

This strategy has implications in virtually every facet of your life. Here, though, we're referring to your being your own advocate about your health.

Initially, you want to make sure that you have been properly diagnosed. If you have any doubts at all, make sure you discuss them with your doctor or consider getting a second opinion. (More about this in Strategy #94.) Once you no longer need to pursue this path, you want to be your own advocate with regard to your prescribed treatment. This is the best way to be a proactive patient.

To use this strategy:

Start by educating yourself about your own diagnosis and treatment.

Here are samples of questions you can ask yourself:

- Am I satisfied that my diagnosis is accurate?

- Do I know enough about my diagnosis, symptoms, medical tests, and treatment?
- Am I comfortable with my medical team?
- Do I feel the need for a second opinion?
- What am I going to do to help myself go through this?

These and other questions will help you to crystallize your advocacy role and determine what steps you may need to take moving forward.

[ ] #36

Monitor the Course of Your Disease

It is almost impossible to predict what you'll experience following your diagnosis. Each person is different. The way you live with your newly diagnosed condition may be as unique as you are.

Be aware of how you're doing as the days and weeks go by. Use strategies to help yourself cope with the "now" as best you can. For example, you may become aware of (and should jot down) strategies that you can use when you're feeling poorly, tired, or lethargic. This may help you to get focused more quickly, and you'll be able to regain control more rapidly. It will also remind you of the need to pace yourself in order to avoid doing too much.

The more you stay on top of the course of your disease, the more active a role you're playing in adjusting to your new reality. You'll also be more aware of any issues that you need to bring to your doctor's attention.

[ ] #37

Turn Unknowns into Next Steps

Life with a chronic illness involves a series of uncertainties.

After your diagnosis, your uncertainties may be at their most intense. You may be apprehensive about the diagnosis itself, the course of the disease, the symptoms you may experience, or your treatments, among other issues.

Unfortunately, regardless of how much may be known about your medical condition, you are still going to feel unsure in the days and weeks following your diagnosis. The one certain thing is that you're going to have to deal with this, and the emotional and physical strain the disease may cause.

Why is it so difficult to deal with uncertainty? We want to know what's going on. Having a sense of what we can anticipate gives us more of a feeling of control. Not knowing what to anticipate, conversely, leads to more of an out-of-control feeling.

Recognize that early on, following your diagnosis with a chronic illness, there may be far more uncertainties than you want. This can be very disconcerting.

As you will frequently read in this book, you're faced with two choices: you can either dwell on or lament this fact, or you can set out to do something about it.

Approach it with the right attitude. Focus on your efforts to learn about your uncertainties and try to reduce the "un" as much as possible.

Try to do everything in your power to attempt to clear up question marks. These question marks are not restricted to what's going on medically in your body. They may include virtually every facet of your life and how it may be affected by your illness.

To use this strategy:

Use your double-column technique in your Coping Notebook. On the left side, pinpoint the specific things you're unsure about. Try to be as specific as you can. Then, on the right side, jot down better ways of dealing with this uncertainty, or who you might consult with in an attempt to clear up any confusion.

[ ] #38
Adapt to Possible Life Changes

Are you apprehensive about the ways your life may change? Most people who are diagnosed are. You may be trying not to think about it. Although this may seem easier (and less frightening), wouldn't it be better if you didn't try so hard to avoid these thoughts and, instead, were better able to deal with them?

What types of changes are we talking about? For example, you may think your lifestyle may change, the goals you previously had for your life may not work, your physical activities may be different, your role in your family may change, or your relationships may change. There are always things you can do to help address or manage these concerns more effectively.

To use this strategy:

Set up a page in your Coping Notebook. Using the double-column technique, on the left side, pinpoint the ways in which you believe your life may change. Try to be as specific as you can. Then, on the right side, jot down ideas for what you can do about each of these, and ways to improve your thinking about the possible life changes.

[ ] #39

Count Your Blessings

There may be many reasons that you start feeling down following your diagnosis. At times, it may be hard to find anything to feel good about. Try to counteract that immediately. Think about the things that you can feel good about (despite your diagnosis). This may seem difficult if you're feeling overwhelmed. However, these are the times when it's even more important to count your blessings!

To use this strategy:

Prepare a list of your blessings. Yes, everyone has some. Let this be a work-in-progress, a list in your Coping Notebook, that you can add to any time an additional positive thought pops into your head. Having this list readily available will help you, especially during those times when you're really feeling down and might have a harder time coming up with something.

Obviously, this is a strategy that you'll be better able to work on when you're feeling good (or even OK). But the idea is for the list you prepare to be there for you when you're not feeling good.

E- What If You Can't Cope?

Nobody's perfect. Although there are many helpful strategies in this chapter (and book), what if there are times when you're so overwhelmed that you just don't have the emotional energy and strength to use them? These strategies can help you deal with that concern.

[ ] #40

Work with Experts

When you feel that you are not able to cope with the hand that has been dealt you, there are experts out there who may be of help. For example, your doctor may suggest you see a mental health professional. Not only would this be a good person for you to talk to, it could also be someone who can guide you in finding better ways of coping with your situation.

Another option is finding support groups in your area. Other avenues to consider include music therapy, yoga, or meditation, just to name a few.

Keep your options open. Recognize when you're not handling things well, and do what you can, speak to whom you can, to help yourself at these times.

To use this strategy:

In your Coping Notebook, write down why you're feeling so overwhelmed. Then write down the steps you're taking to find an expert who can help you with what you're going through. (See Strategy #110 for additional information about this.) Finally, write down the specific things you want to get help with when you connect with your expert.

[ ] #41

Consider Medication to Help You Cope

You know yourself best. You know how you feel emotionally. You also know what strategies you have attempted, up to this point, to try to improve the way you feel.

However, what if you feel so overwhelmed by your diagnosis that it is interfering with your ability to function, to the point that you're not able to focus on any strategies? You may want to consider medication as an assist. That's what it's there for.

There are effective medications available that can alleviate the intense emotional discomfort you may be experiencing. Discuss this with your doctor. Don't hesitate to mention that you're considering something temporarily to help you in the early stages (or any stage when you think it's necessary) of coping with your diagnosis.

Obviously, you want to make sure that any medications you consider are compatible with your ongoing treatment plan. This will best be decided by your physician (or a consultation with a psychiatrist may be suggested).

In either case, know that the goal is not for you to be on this type of medication long-term. Remember, you're using medication for one reason, and that is to get back to the point where using your strategies will help you cope.

WHAT'S NEXT?

This chapter has focused on helping you understand both your emotional reactions and the facts about your condition. Knowledge, acceptance, and perspective are all part of building resilience. The next chapter will guide you toward greater acceptance, equipping you with strategies to work through the emotional ups and downs that inevitably accompany chronic illness.

CHAPTER 3

I Need to Accept and Adapt

Accept your diagnosis? This might elicit a sarcastic laugh. The last thing that most people want to do when they've been diagnosed with a chronic illness is to simply accept it. They want to fight it. They want to deny it. They want to prove that it's incorrect. They're angry about it. They want to believe that they're still healthy. As you read in the last chapter, this is all part of the first four stages of grieving.

But the stage we're talking about now is the fifth stage: acceptance.

Have you heard of the Serenity Prayer? To paraphrase: the goal is for you to have the serenity (or calmness) to accept things that you cannot change, the courage to change the things you can, and the wisdom to know the difference. Isn't that the goal of accepting your diagnosis?

Acceptance doesn't mean surrender. It's not about liking your diagnosis or pretending it doesn't hurt. It's about facing reality honestly so that you can begin to regain a sense of control and move forward.

The goal is not to embrace your illness as something positive, but to acknowledge it as part of your life. Acceptance opens the door to coping, evolving, and reclaiming your life

And now, on to acceptance.

A- Move Towards Acceptance

So, how do you get started in the process of acceptance? Consider the following strategies as a starting point. Once again, remember that you don't have to do all of them. Select the ones that make the most sense to you.

[ ] #42

Accept and Embrace Your "New Normal"

Yes, your life will be different following your diagnosis. Sure, there may be (many) times when you wish you could go back to things the way they used to be. We all wish that from time to time. Unfortunately, the reality is that no one can. We can only try to move forward in a positive way.

However, this doesn't mean that your life is only going to be bad. Not only can it be good, in some ways it may even be better. (And it's up to you to help to make that happen.)

With your diagnosis comes the understanding that certain characteristics of who you are have changed. This becomes your new normal. But it doesn't mean that you're a totally different person. There are still many aspects of your life that are the same as they were before your diagnosis.

You want to put less and less energy into lamenting the loss of your life as it was. So, your aim is to accept your diagnosis, and make the best of it, while you learn how to better deal with your new normal.

What should you do? Keep telling yourself, "*It is what it is. I know I can be strong and do whatever it is I have to do.*" You want to assimilate this new normal into the person that you've always been. As much as you may not want to accept this, even getting emotional about it, your new normal is the way it is. Your goal is to accept, cope, and move forward.

[ ] #43

See Yourself as a Person First, Patient Second

Before being diagnosed, you probably never had a reason to distinguish between these two labels. But now you have a chronic illness. So now, you feel like a patient.

Here is a better way of looking at it:

If you go to the doctor, you are a patient. If you go to the hospital, you are a patient. But you are still a person who happens to be a patient.

The rest of the time, you are a person. Don't let your diagnosis "depersonalize" you!

To use this strategy:

Make a conscious effort to use language that reflects your identity. Write in your Coping Notebook: *"I am a person who has [condition], not just a patient."* Surround yourself with activities, people, and goals that remind you of your identity beyond illness.

[ ] #44

Prepare for a Tug-of-War

As you start working on acceptance, you'll find that there will be more and more snippets of time when you feel better. Then something will happen that will make you unhappy again. Prepare for that- it's a normal part of learning to adjust to your diagnosis.

Don't worry that these unhappy times mean that you'll never be happy again. Instead, be prepared for this emotional tug-of-war. It is a very common part of the acceptance process.

To use this strategy:

Talk to yourself. Remember that you can choose to be an active tug-of-war participant. Keep fighting back, get yourself to focus on thoughts that are realistic and positive when the negative, unhappy thoughts threaten to pull you down.

The more you do this, the more you'll gain confidence in your ability to straighten your thinking out in a more positive direction… and win the tug-of-war!

[ ] #45

Don't Blame Yourself for Your Condition

You may feel as though your body let you down. You may feel that you didn't follow proper, healthy steps to avoid what you're currently going through. Why dwell on that?

There are many different factors which may have come together to lead to your diagnosis. Some of them may have to do with your actions (or lack thereof). More likely though, life just happens! Why blame yourself for this (even if, in any way, you contributed)? It's an enormous waste of time and energy. Will it change the diagnosis? No!

Put your energy into helping your body, and your mind, instead of knocking yourself down.

To use this strategy:

Whenever self-blaming thoughts pop into your head, respond to them with this mantra: *"It is what it is, and I'm going to make the best of it!"* Write this mantra in your Coping Notebook and repeat it daily until it becomes automatic. That's positive, that's realistic, and that's constructive.

[ ] #46

Remember Who You Still Are

Other than your condition, symptoms, and lifestyle changes necessitated by it, aren't you still the same person you were before the diagnosis? You still like the same flavor of ice cream, watch the same television programs, and read the same books.

There are so many ways that you're still the same person. Your condition is just a new wrinkle. Yes, it may be a difficult one, but it is part of the overall mosaic of who you are.

To use this strategy:

Make a two-column list in your Coping Notebook. On one side, write down what has changed. On the other side, write down what has stayed the same. Review this list if you find yourself having difficulty with this concept.

[ ] #47

Embrace Your Whole Self—Mind and Body

Focus on accepting more than just your physical symptoms. Focus on accepting the totality of who you are. Work on accepting your emotions and thoughts, not only the physical aspects of your illness.

It's understandable at first to obsess about the way you're feeling physically. Sure, you may be frightened, worrying about the implications of your prognosis.

But as time goes on and you receive treatment, you'll remember that there is more to your life than just physical symptoms. Anticipate anxiety, depression, and other emotional reactions, and be prepared to put the same amount of effort into dealing with them as you do with your physical symptoms.

To use this strategy:

Set aside a few minutes each day to check in with your mind, not just your body. Ask yourself questions like: *"What feelings am I experiencing? What thoughts keep returning?"* Write these answers in your Coping Notebook. Then, next to them, note what helped—whether it was talking with someone, journaling, relaxation, or simply naming the feeling. Over time, you'll build a personal guide to managing emotional acceptance, just as you track your physical progress.

[ ] #48

Let Go of the Need for Total Control

This may sound like simple common sense, but the people who have the hardest time adjusting after diagnoses are often those who are so used to being in control, and need to be in control, that they have a hard time when they're not in control. When that control disappears, the contrast can feel unbearable.

No one can be in control all the time. Yes, you want to control as much as you can. Most people do. But when you can't control everything, aim to accept that. Learn to go with the flow.

Concentrate on the things you can control, instead of dwelling on things you can't. That will help restore a sense of control more quickly.

To use this strategy:

Each day, list one thing you can control and one thing you cannot. Then focus your effort only on the first item. Over time, this practice will retrain your mind to let go of the rest.

[ ] #49

Meet Challenges with Resolve

You're going to go through a lot of different experiences, reactions, annoyances, and discomforts in your life following your diagnosis. Expect them. However, don't be put off by them. You can get through them.

Yes, you can get through this and even be happy. (What a concept!) This usually has less to do with the condition itself and more to do with the way you think about it, cope with it, and strengthen your life.

To use this strategy:

Take the action approach. When you feel a certain way, ask yourself how you can get past it, rather than lamenting that you have to go through it. If you are unable to come up with answers, reach out to significant others or professionals for guidance. Write down approaches that worked, so you can reuse them next time.

[ ] #50

Accept Setbacks as Part of the Journey

One of the hardest truths about chronic illness is that progress is rarely a straight line. You might be feeling better for a while, only to face a flare-up or new limitation. That can be discouraging—unless you expect it.

Setbacks don't erase your progress; they're simply part of the journey. Think of coping like hiking a mountain trail: sometimes the path is smooth, sometimes it's rocky, and sometimes you need to pause and catch your breath. Even those pauses are part of getting to the top.

To use this strategy:

When a setback occurs, begin by naming it for what it is—a temporary pause, not a failure. Remind yourself of times in the past when you've rebounded and use those memories as evidence that you can do it again. Return to your most reliable coping tools, such as relaxation techniques, journaling, or reaching out to a friend, rather than searching for something entirely new in the moment. Finally, choose one small, manageable action you can take today to start moving forward again. Even a single step will help you regain momentum and rebuild confidence.

[ ] #51

Hold Onto and Adapt Your Dreams

Are you supposed to abandon your dreams because of your diagnosis? Some people fear they must, but this isn't true.

Don't allow yourself to believe that, because of your diagnosis, you must abandon your dreams.

In some cases, the path to those dreams may have to be adjusted. In other cases, some of your goals may need to change because of the reality of your situation. But it's far better to adapt to the changes, maintain your dreams, and even add new ones, than to not have them, or to let them go.

To use this strategy:

Ask yourself what you want to accomplish in your life. What are your dreams? Write your answers in your Coping Notebook. Then, separate those goals that are realistic from those that are not. (Don't despair-- sometimes goals that are currently unrealistic may become more realistic in time.) As you focus more on those goals that are currently realistic, jot down the steps you might take to head in the right direction.

[ ] #52

Understand That Acceptance Takes Time

A very common feeling following a diagnosis is the desire to get back to living your life the way you did before the diagnosis… as quickly as possible!

Well, it may not happen quickly, but it can happen! It will involve acceptance and adjustment to all of the changes that are taking place in your life. Keep reminding yourself: these changes take time, and acceptance follows gradually.

But don't put time pressures on yourself. Obviously, acceptance is not an overnight thing (even though you'd like it to be!). Acknowledge the obstacles and work on your coping strategies. You'll get there.

To use this strategy:

Use your support team to help you to get through those periods when you feel that acceptance and happiness are more elusive. Record milestones—however small—in your Coping Notebook to remind yourself that progress is happening.

[ ] #53

See Yourself in a Positive Light

Before you were diagnosed, you probably had a picture in your mind of who you were. You knew how you did things, how you handled things, and what you were all about. But be honest with yourself: Did you always handle everything perfectly?

Now you've been diagnosed with a chronic illness, and you may be having a hard time dealing with things that have changed. So, what should you do?

Picture the way you want to be ... realistically. Recognize that many things about you are still the same as they were. For those things that have changed, think about how you can fit this into your new normal. For everything that you can't do, think about something that you can do, or something new that you can learn to do. Give yourself the opportunity to grow and to feel good about some of these changes.

For some people, the thought of being different is scary. It's better, though, to think of it as a challenge, one in which you can enjoy the things about you that are the same and grow to feel better about the new aspects of yourself shaped by your diagnosis.

Be positive. If you have difficulty doing this, reach out to someone (family member, friend, or mental health professional) who can help support your efforts.

Don't let your diagnosis define who you are. Focus on redefining yourself ... as you choose.

To use this strategy:

Write a description of your "positive self" in your Coping Notebook—who you want to be and how you want to live. Make sure it's a realistic description. Revisit this page in your notebook often, especially during difficult days.

[ ] #54

Strengthen Resilience Through Gratitude

Living with illness can easily shift your focus toward what has changed or what feels diminished—energy, routines, or independence. Gratitude offers a counterbalance, helping you notice what continues to bring comfort, meaning, and joy. This doesn't mean denying hardship. Instead, gratitude helps you create a fuller, more balanced perspective, reminding you that good moments and sustaining resources are still present alongside the challenges.

Research has shown that people who practice gratitude regularly experience greater emotional stability, reduced stress, and even improved physical well-being. By making gratitude part of your daily routine, you train your mind to look for positives, which can lighten your mood and give you greater strength to cope when times are tough. Gratitude also deepens connections with others, since recognizing and expressing appreciation builds warmth and mutual support.

To use this strategy:

Each day, pause to reflect on specific things you feel grateful for, whether large or small—a meaningful conversation, a comforting meal, or even the simple fact that you made it through the day. Write them down in your Coping Notebook to create a growing record of positives you can revisit when you're struggling. When possible, share your gratitude with others; a thank-you note, a spoken word of appreciation, or a kind gesture reinforces the habit and strengthens your relationships. Over time, this practice not only shifts your focus away from what illness may have taken but also helps you build resilience by drawing energy from what remains good in your life.

[ ] #55

Accept ... and Then Adapt

Why is it so important to accept your diagnosis? Because acceptance allows you to begin adapting. Adapting means adjusting to a new situation or condition. In your case, this is your new normal. You're adapting by identifying the changes that you need to make to live with your chronic illness and learning how to implement these changes in your lifestyle.

To use this strategy:

Start thinking of any changes you may need to make. Write them down in your Coping Notebook. You can add to the list as new needs arise. It doesn't mean you have to make all changes at once.

Make another list of the things you'll be able to continue to do, despite your illness. Certain things may require some changes, limitations, or alterations. But many activities may remain unaffected. The goal is to combine new aspects of your life necessitated by your diagnosis with the old aspects of your life that you're still able to enjoy.

Work to create a healthy balance between old and new. It will help you to feel like yourself, and you'll know you're accepting, and adapting!

B - Practical Strategies for Acceptance

Even as you accept your condition, you won't always remain fully in acceptance. New symptoms, changes in treatment, or life events may push you back into earlier stages of adjustment.

Don't be put off by that. Anticipate it. Then just go into coping mode to guide yourself back to acceptance once again.

Just as your medical condition fluctuates, so too will your emotional response. Recognize these ups and downs as part of the process, not a sign of failure.

[ ] #56

Learn and Respect Your Limits

One of the realities following your diagnosis is that you may not be able to do as much as you used to in certain areas of your life. Acceptance of this may take time, but it is important.

It is important to know when to push yourself and when not to. If you overdo, you may experience negative consequences.

Pacing is key. There may be times when you need to rest, possibly more than you ever have before. Resting will help you recharge so that you can maximize the things that you are able to do (and want to do). See Strategy #135 for more information about this.

To use this strategy:

Write down examples of when you've overdone it and how it affected you. Use these notes to identify your boundaries and adjust your pacing.

[ ] #57

Be Patient with the Process

Are you someone who feels you need to learn everything about your condition right away, or accept it immediately? That urgency is understandable, but it often backfires. Acceptance is not something that can be rushed. It requires patience.

Look at acceptance as being a destination and try to be comfortable during the ride. This will help you make the most of your efforts to learn about your illness while also living your life. Keeping this balance is essential.

To use this strategy:

Permit yourself to move at a natural pace. Set aside short, specific times to read, learn, or reflect on your illness, and balance those with times devoted to ordinary routines and pleasures. When frustration builds, pause and write down one small sign of progress in your Coping Notebook. Schedule breaks to rest or engage in activities that bring you comfort, so the process of acceptance develops alongside—not in place of—your daily life.

[ ] #58

Know When to Try… and When to Take a Break

Many of the strategies you've been reading about have to do with things you should try to do. But what if you feel guilty because you don't feel like doing anything? You may worry that this means that you'll never accept your diagnosis, never cope with it, and never find happiness. Nothing could be further from the truth.

You can't work all the time. And you can't (and shouldn't) focus on coping strategies nonstop.

There are times when you just need to take a break! So, do it! Relax, rest, or choose something self-indulgent. Whatever you do, the goal is to clear your head and enable you to effectively resume working on the things you need to work on … especially acceptance.

To use this strategy:

Create a "break list" of activities that refresh you. Add to your list as you think of new or different ideas. Refer to this list when you feel guilty about resting, as a reminder that breaks are not wasted time but an essential part of coping.

[ ] #59

Stop Yourself from Obsessing Over Your Illness

It's certainly understandable to think about your diagnosis and all of its implications. It's also appropriate to think about what you're doing as part of your self-improvement program.

However, when you're thinking about it constantly and unable to focus elsewhere, then you're obsessing. This can crowd out all the other things you might need ... and want ... to think about.

To use this strategy:

Your goal is to redirect your thinking to something other than your illness. Some ideas include:

- Picture a big red stop sign. Then, immediately redirect yourself to something else.
- Snap a rubber band on your wrist. (Gently!) The momentary "tingle" distracts you long enough to shift your focus.
- Pre-plan distraction strategies and write them in your Coping Notebook for those times when you find yourself obsessing. (See Strategy #8.)

Sometimes you may choose to be more aggressive. For example, in addition to picturing a big red stop sign, you might say to yourself (or out loud, if there's no one around), "Stop that!" This isn't anger. It's intensity- a way to break the cycle.

Sometimes "forbidding" yourself to obsess makes it even harder to stop. As an alternative, you may want to give yourself a limited, set amount of time to think about your diagnosis, or any related issues or questions. (More about this in the next strategy.)

[ ] #60

Benefit from Regular "Chair Time"

Despite your efforts at accepting your condition, there may be times when you just can't stop yourself from thinking about it. You may find yourself obsessing over your diagnosis, its implications, or any of the symptoms that you may experience. You may even find yourself feeling sorry for yourself. All of this is not unusual. The more you fight the thoughts, the stronger they can feel.

That's where "chair time" comes in. It's scheduled time you intentionally set aside to think about anything about your condition that just doesn't stop popping into your mind.

To use this strategy:

Choose one or two specific times a day to allow yourself five minutes of "chair time," during which you focus only on your illness and related concerns. The chair is just a symbol—you can do this in bed, while walking, or anywhere else.

Use this time to write down your thoughts, questions, or worries, giving them a place outside your mind. At the end of those five minutes, stop deliberately—get up, walk away, and turn to something else. If thoughts about your illness arise later, remind yourself they can wait until your next designated "chair time." With regular practice, this method reduces intrusive thinking and frees your mind (thankfully) to focus on other things.

[ ] #61

Hold On to Hope

Following your diagnosis, have there ever been times when you felt like giving up? If so, you're not alone. This is a common experience for many people.

When might this occur? Possibly, soon after your diagnosis. Or maybe after some time has gone by and you're having difficulty accomplishing certain things. In short, anyone can encounter an emotional roadblock due to the twists and turns of living with a chronic condition. But you want (and need) to keep on going. Hope fuels resilience, determination, and the will to keep moving forward.

Recognize that these feelings come and go, and while they can be overpowering, they are temporary. The more intensely you feel like giving up, the more important it is to reach out to people who can support you when you need them. Their support can stabilize you and help you get back on your feet.

To use this strategy:

If the urge to give up feels overwhelming, open your Coping Notebook. Write down the specific thoughts and feelings you are experiencing in that moment. Next, list at least one small, constructive action you can take right away—such as making a phone call, taking a short walk, or practicing a relaxation exercise.

On another page, create a list of people you can reach out to when hope feels distant, including family, friends, or professionals. Keep their contact information handy. Each time you use this strategy, review your notes to remind yourself that hopelessness has occurred before and it will pass. These written reminders, combined with small steps forward, can help anchor you when your motivation feels weakest.

WHAT'S NEXT?

Acceptance is not the end of your journey—it's the foundation for what comes next. The next chapter will help you move beyond acceptance, with strategies to get back on your feet, re-engage with life, and keep building momentum as you move forward with strength.

CHAPTER 4

I Need to Find My Pace and Priorities

Getting a diagnosis may have knocked you down—but it doesn't mean you have to stay down. In the first three chapters, you've learned strategies to help you deal with the shock, make sense of your reactions, and begin accepting your new reality. Now it's time to take the next step: finding practical ways to get back on your feet and re-enter life, even with illness as part of it.

The goal isn't perfection or recreating your "old" life—it's progress. That means focusing on what you *can* do, learning to pace yourself, and rebuilding confidence little by little. In this chapter, you'll learn practical strategies to help you restore balance, build resilience, and regain momentum. These tools will support you as you create a new version of your life that feels both possible and meaningful.

A- First Steps Back

The first steps in getting back on your feet involve starting small and focusing on what you *can* do, not what you can't. You may not be able to return to the exact life you had before your diagnosis, but you can begin creating a new balance that works for you. This section introduces strategies designed to help you shift from reacting to your illness to actively taking steps forward. Each one will encourage you to build confidence, regain independence, and strengthen your foundation for progress.

[ ] #62

Be Proactive Instead of Reactive

Are you typically proactive or reactive? What exactly does that mean?

There are many different adjectives you can use to describe how you feel and what you go through following the diagnosis of a chronic illness. You may feel overwhelmed, devastated, terrified, panicky or hopeless? These are all reactive words.

The goal is to shift to becoming proactive ... to focus on how to move forward, rather than just dwelling on how you're reacting to the diagnosis.

Yes, of course, you'll have reactive feelings at times. But you don't want to stay there. Progress begins when you start doing things to help yourself and move forward. It's up to you how long you allow yourself to remain stuck in reaction before choosing to take proactive steps.

To use this strategy:

When you notice reactive thoughts or feelings, write them in your Coping Notebook. Acknowledge them honestly. Then try to immediately respond to them by reminding yourself to be proactive.

Then, beneath each one, respond with a proactive statement such as: "What can I do about this right now?" If the answer is "nothing at this moment," set it aside and redirect your energy toward something you *can* do. Over time, this practice strengthens your ability to recover and regain control more quickly.

[ ] #63

Determine Your Self-Improvement Pace

It's important to determine your own pace. Some people want to work as fast as they can. Others may be hesitant to move too fast; they may want to move more slowly to make sure they stick with their program. By being deliberate about your pace, you're more likely to benefit from your self-improvement efforts. Setting your own pace also prevents burnout, increases consistency, and makes your progress sustainable.

To use this strategy:

In your Coping Notebook, jot down notes about what pace feels realistic for you. Be realistic and honest in answering the following two questions:

- How much time do you want to spend each day on your self-improvement program?
- When are the best times for you to work on them?

Use these answers to guide how many strategies you want to work on each day and for how long.

Your answers may change from day to day, or in general. That's fine. But remember, working at a pace that's realistic for you is the best way to stick with your program and keep moving forward.

[ ] #64

Do What You Can Yourself

An unfortunate consequence of the diagnosis of a chronic illness is a feeling of dependency. You may feel dependent on the medical profession. You may worry about depending more on your family to help, or take care of, you.

Yes, you will have an ongoing, helpful relationship with both your medical team and your family. Research shows that the more you do for yourself, the better you feel about yourself and your life. Taking even small steps for yourself helps you feel more in control and less helpless.

To use this strategy:

Make a list of all the things that you currently do for yourself. Then make a list of things that you may not currently do but feel you can and should do. Develop a plan to implement these things into your daily routine.

Although there may be times when you feel overwhelmed or may be physically unable to do these things, by having them on your list, they'll be something for you to aim to accomplish. Won't you feel good moving items from the "don't" to the "do" side?

There may be certain things on the "don't" side that you won't be able to do, or choose not to do (realistically, of course!). As long as you're being sensible and honest with yourself, don't worry about those. Focus more on your "do" side.

[ ] #65

Prioritize

Do you know what the priorities are in your life? Most people don't think about this because deep down, they know what they are. But your diagnosis may have changed all that.

Following your diagnosis, you may find that your physical and emotional resources occasionally feel limited. In other words, you may not always be able to do as much as you did.

So, you'll want to make sure that you maximize your abilities when you can. You'll want to focus your physical and emotional energy on the most important tasks and activities that you need to complete. This is an important reason to prioritize.

Ironically, before the diagnosis of a chronic illness, taking care of one's health is often fairly low on the priority list. But now, caring for your physical condition will be an important foundation for being able to do more of the things you want.

To use this strategy:

Make a list of your priorities as they exist right now. Indicate today's date. Keep it in your Coping Notebook. Check your list regularly—not only to stay focused, but also to see if anything needs to move up or down.

Make sure that your health is always high on the list and write at least one action step for each priority.

[ ] #66

Be Prepared for Feelings and Fluctuations

As you make progress in dealing with your chronic illness, you may start feeling better. But that doesn't mean that you'll always feel good. (Then again, did you always feel good before your diagnosis?)

Some of your initial feelings may return. It's hard to predict when this will happen. But you're better off anticipating these fluctuations. In this way, you can use your coping strategies to get back on track when they do happen.

To use this strategy:

In your Coping Notebook, track both the times when you feel you're making progress and the times when you don't. When do your feelings fluctuate? Write what triggers these fluctuations, what helps you bounce back, and what indications you'll notice that show you that you're improving again. These notes will remind you that setbacks are temporary, not permanent.

[ ] #67

Find Your Balance

Everybody needs balance in their lives. Feeling out of balance is sure to make you feel unsettled and uncomfortable.

What creates balance for you is as unique as your fingerprint. Following a diagnosis, you may not immediately know what will help you feel in balance—it often takes thought and experimentation.

You won't learn how to improve your balance all at once. In fact, it may take time following your diagnosis to become more confident in knowing your balance. Over time, you'll become more comfortable recognizing what balance feels like for you.

If it hasn't happened yet, remind yourself that balance takes time to develop, and each step you take brings you closer.

To use this strategy:

In your Coping Notebook, track the differences between times you feel comfortable and times you don't. Write down the circumstances, activities, people, or routines that contribute to balance, and those that disrupt it. Notice that this may change from day to day or even moment to moment. By reviewing your notes, you'll begin to recognize patterns and discover your own formula for balance.

B- Good Tools To Use

In addition to the first steps you've just worked on, there are some broader tools that can guide your progress in almost any area of life. These strategies are practical skills you can apply again and again. Think of them as building blocks: they not only help you get back on your feet now but also give you a framework you can rely on whenever you face new challenges.

[ ] #68

Identify the Specific Ways That Your Diagnosis Affects You

Each person is unique. Your response to your diagnosis will be unique as well. The variety of ways people respond to a diagnosis includes the physical impact that the disease may have (obviously), the impact on your family, as well as any emotional, financial, vocational, and social impact.

Recognizing these different effects gives you a clearer picture of what you're dealing with and where to focus your energy.

To use this strategy:

As you work to cope with your diagnosis, write down any of the possible specific things that you may be overwhelmed by, including:

- Learning about your disease, its treatment, its symptoms, and its impact
- How your body may change
- How much you need to learn
- The changes you need to make in your lifestyle
- The new people who will be part of your life (e.g., your treatment team)
- How your friendships may change (who will continue to be supportive, and who may not understand)
- The impact the disease may have on your emotions
- How to maintain a positive mental attitude, despite your illness

Refer back to other strategies in this book that match each area you've listed and note the strategy numbers in your Coping Notebook. Then begin by writing specific steps you can take to address them. The following three strategies will help you get started.

[ ] #69

Separate What You Can Control from What You Can't

It's important to be able to separate those factors, issues, and problems in your life and your illness that you can control from those that you can't.

For those things that you can control, start working on developing an action plan, including strategies that can make a difference. (The next two strategies can be helpful with this.)

We cannot control (or even do something about) everything that may occur because of a diagnosis. But there are still ways to cope more effectively—even when change isn't possible—by working on your thinking and response.

To use this strategy:

In your Coping Notebook, make a double-column list: list on one side the items that you can address, change, or improve. On the other side, write those things that you can't change and need to accept. This will help you to determine what to focus on and what strategies can help.

Examples of things that you can do something about are the way you eat, the way you comply with treatment regimens (including medications), who you spend time with (e.g., minimizing contact with people who have an adverse impact on you), pacing yourself differently to conserve your strength, etc.

An example of something that you cannot do anything about is having the disease!

Then, take each of the items that you've written and set up a separate page indicating the steps you can take (either to do something about it, or to work on your thinking about it).

[ ] #70

Pinpoint the Things You Want to Work On

An important step in any self-improvement program is pinpointing the specific areas you will target. Pinpointing is different than identifying or distinguishing, as discussed in the previous strategy. Pinpointing helps you determine exactly what you want to improve.

There are many areas that may be important to you in your life following a diagnosis. These may include improving your ability to deal with your emotional reactions, coping with physical symptoms, reducing your anger or fear, dealing with changes in your family, and communicating with your doctor. By pinpointing any of the factors that are important to you, you're in a better position to work on them.

To use this strategy:

In your Coping Notebook, write every answer you can think of that completes the following sentence:

I would like to improve or better deal with ....

Make sure that your answers are clear-cut and unambiguous.

Each answer starts the process of pinpointing what you want or need to work on. Use the double-column technique here: write an answer to the above sentence completion on the left side of the page, your goal, and on the right, the steps you may take to work on this.

Now imagine someone else reading your answer. Would that person immediately understand exactly what you want to work on? If you're confident that they would, great! You're ready to start working on this item. If not, however, ask yourself how you could make your answer even more clear and specific, so this other person would "get it." Now you're pinpointing, which will help you get ready for the next strategy-setting goals.

[ ] #71

Set Clear Goals for Your Self-Improvement Efforts

You'll want to establish specific goals for any pinpointed item that you want to tackle.

A very important rule for doing this is that you want your goals to be precise, observable, and measurable. For example, it would be far more accurate and precise to say, "I'm going to include a 30-minute 're-energizing' nap each afternoon, between 3 and 4 o'clock, in my schedule" than to say, "I'm going to rest more." A goal is observable if someone can see what you're doing, and measurable if you can clearly confirm that it's been done.

To use this strategy:

On a new page in your Coping Notebook, write down one of your pinpointed items as a target for goal-setting. Then indicate the following answers about that item.

- What would I like to improve or deal with better?
- Why is this a problem?
- What goal(s) would I like to set? (Be sure your goals are clear, precise, and measurable—clear enough that anyone reading them would immediately know what you intend to accomplish.)
- What strategies can I use in an attempt to achieve my goal(s)? (You can use any of the strategies described in this book, or other strategies that you may find helpful.)
- What is the step-by-step, detailed action plan, indicating exactly what I'm going to do? (If you find that certain steps are more difficult to accomplish, break them down into smaller steps.)

Track your progress regularly and adjust your steps as necessary, but always keep your desired end result in mind. Just knowing that you're working on these items will help you to know that you're moving in the right direction. (Use your notebook to continue this work for additional items you've pinpointed, or additional strategies you're going to use.)

And remember to celebrate each goal you check off—you'll be able to look back and see tangible proof of your progress.

WHAT'S NEXT?

You now have strategies that can help you regain momentum and start rebuilding your life. The next chapter focuses on putting these skills into action during treatment—so you can strengthen your resilience and take an active role in your care.

CHAPTER 5

I Need to Be an Active Treatment Partner

One of the most important ways to move forward after your diagnosis is to become an active participant in your treatment. That means learning as much as you can about your body, your symptoms, and your treatment plan. The more you know, the more ownership you'll have over your health journey. This chapter introduces strategies to help you play a proactive role in your treatment. In the next chapter, we'll focus on working more effectively with your healthcare team.

A- Dealing with Your Treatment

One of the frustrating feelings that people have when they're diagnosed is the sense that their condition is controlling them. This is not true ... unless you let it. How do you let it happen? You don't do anything. You're not proactive. You don't explore what you can do to help your symptoms.

It's true that it's not your choice to have this condition. But it is your choice how much you allow it to control you.

So, learn about your illness. Learn what the symptoms are, but more importantly, learn what you can do about them. Learn about the treatments- medical methods, medications, physical therapy, and more.

Most important, learn what you can do to support those treatments. That's your job.

Treatment protocols can contain many components. In this section, you'll find strategies to show what you can do to play an active role in your treatment.

[ ] #72

Keep Track of All Treatment Information

Discussing your treatment plan with your physician is one of the first things you'll do following your diagnosis. Make sure you understand everything you're told.

It can be very helpful to have all information about your prescribed treatment in one place. This makes it easy to refer to, helps you to keep track of exactly what you need to do, and gives you a place to note additions, changes, or results. Your treatment may involve one approach, or there may be several components- making it even more important to track everything carefully.

To use this strategy:

In your Coping Notebook, set up a treatment page. Record details such as:

- What treatment was prescribed for you
- Who prescribed it and when
- The goal of the treatment
- What exactly do you have to do
- Whether the treatment is helping
- Questions for your doctor

Keep your treatment page or your Coping Notebook with you at all appointments and write down everything you need to remember. When you get home, add more details, including who said what, when, and where.

Any modifications to be made in your treatment plan can also be included on these pages. Upcoming strategies will give you other ideas about how best to do this.

Keep this information up to date. Not only will it help you when you go to your doctors' appointments, it will also be invaluable if you see new doctors.

[ ] #73

Play an Active Role in Your Care

As noted earlier, your doctors will explain the components of your treatment. They'll discuss their role. It's also important to focus on your role. Your job is to be an active participant in your treatment.

Don't just be a blind follower. Being an active participant involves more than just doing what your medical team tells you.

To use this strategy:

On the treatment page in your Coping Notebook (see Strategy #72), add the specific things you can do to be an active participant in your treatment. For example:

- Ask questions.
- Offer suggestions.
- Give feedback.
- Comply with recommendations.
- Keep records.

Keep adding to your list as you learn of additional things you can do.

Show your doctors that you care about yourself and about what they're trying to do to help you. This doesn't mean that you have to control everything. A good doctor-patient relationship is built on partnership, teamwork, and communication—neither side controls everything.

[ ] #74

Use Apps and Technology Tools to Stay Organized

Managing an illness often means keeping track of a lot—medications, appointments, test results, and instructions from different providers. That can feel overwhelming. Technology can make this easier. Tools like medication reminder apps, secure patient portals, telehealth visits, or even simple calendar alerts can act like a helper, keeping you organized and making sure less slips through the cracks.

To use this strategy:

Ask your care team if they recommend any apps or tools for tracking your medications or symptoms. Set reminders on your phone or calendar for important routines, like taking your meds or getting to appointments. Use your patient portal to check results or send non-urgent questions to your doctor. If you prefer digital notes, keep them alongside your Coping Notebook so everything stays in one place.

[ ] #75

Use Your Question/Answer Page

As you move forward, questions about your illness and treatment will naturally come up—sometimes at unexpected times, like in the middle of the night, or when you least expect it. If you don't write them down, they may slip away, and you might forget to ask at your next appointment.

Collecting these questions—and the answers—gives you a comprehensive, reliable resource that prevents confusion, keeps you engaged, and ensures your appointments are more productive. It also helps you see your own progress as your list of unanswered questions gradually turns into answers you can rely on.

To use this strategy:

In your Coping Notebook, use the Question/Answer page that you initially set up as part of Strategy #19. Write down every question that comes to mind, especially anything you don't understand, feel uncertain about, or want clarified—and leave space to record the answers.

Keep adding to your list of questions as they occur. Bring this page with you to each appointment so you can track your progress, get answers as they arise, and keep your treatment moving forward.

[ ] #76

Make Sure You Comply with Your Treatment Protocol

Treatment is the most important practical consideration following your diagnosis. What is going to be done to get your disease under control ... and help you to feel better? Your doctor(s) will be working to figure out what treatment protocol makes the most sense for you, your condition, and your symptoms.

Once a program is in place, make sure you follow it. Sure, you can ask questions about it and report any problems you encounter. But, what's the point of getting recommendations and then not following them? Non-compliance may signal a bigger problem such as denial, self-destructive behavior, or rebellion—and this needs to be addressed quickly before your condition worsens.

If you have a problem with compliance, or sticking to your program, admit it to yourself…quickly- and then do something about it. Ask yourself why you're not complying. What's holding you back? Identifying what may be interfering with effective compliance is the first step toward change.

Discuss any compliance issues with your doctor. If your doctor is unable to help you, or you're afraid to admit it, speak to a healthcare professional who can help you understand why this is happening and what you can do to get back on track.

[ ] #77

Know Your Patient Rights

Being a patient can sometimes feel like you've lost control. Hospitals and clinics may seem like places with their own rules, and it's easy to feel like you have no say. But knowing your rights helps you feel steadier and more involved. You have the right to ask questions until you understand, to see your medical records, to get a second opinion, and to ask for reasonable changes at work or school. These rights don't make every problem go away, but they can keep you from feeling powerless and remind you that you are an important part of your care.

To use this strategy:

Find out what patient rights apply where you live—for example, by looking up a "Patient Bill of Rights." Write down the ones that matter most to you in your Coping Notebook. If something doesn't feel right, look at your notes and use them as a reminder to ask—politely but firmly—until you're clear. Remember, speaking up for yourself isn't being difficult. It's simply taking care of yourself.

[ ] #78

Become a Self-Care Expert

The more confident you are in your ability to care for yourself, the better you will deal with your illness. Confidence in self-care improves your quality of life and strengthens your sense of control.

Research shows that the more of an active role you take in your health care, the better the outcome. This is why becoming a self-care expert is so important.

You want to be involved in as many facets of your self-care as possible. Because you've been diagnosed with a chronic illness, you want to do everything you can to help yourself. This is you investing in yourself.

This is a process- but it doesn't mean you need to do everything alone.

This may involve more effort early on. The good news is that as you live with it, much of your effort will become second nature. Early on, though, it's important to stay on top of as much as possible.

Make your doctor a partner in your care. But remember that the primary responsibility is yours. You don't want to depend entirely upon your doctor.

To use this strategy:

In your Coping Notebook, create a Self-Care Log. Record activities such as monitoring symptoms, checking vitals (temperature, pulse, blood pressure, respiration rate), and making lifestyle changes (diet, exercise, rest). Note when you need to call your doctor and record what you learn from those calls. Review your log weekly to see what's becoming second nature and where you still need to focus.

[ ] #79

Know Your Medications

Unfortunately, many chronic illnesses require medication as part of treatment. But fortunately, many symptoms can be successfully controlled or improved with the right medications.

Think of it this way: if you really want to regain some control over your condition (and your life), it makes sense to know as much as you can about any medications that you're prescribed.

To use this strategy:

In your Coping Notebook, set up a separate page for each medication you're prescribed. Include the following information:

- Medication name and dosage
- Purpose of the medication
- How long it should take to work
- How and when to take it (e.g., with food, before meals, after meals)
- Potential side effects (including what to do if they occur, and when to contact your doctor
- Any potentially harmful interactions with other medications or substances
- Any other important details

If you're unsure about anything, ask your doctor, nurse, pharmacist, or other healthcare professionals to clarify.

[ ] #80

Be Prepared to Deal with Side Effects

All medications have side effects (though you won't necessarily experience them). As unpleasant as side effects may be, remind yourself: if a medication is powerful enough to cause side effects, it's also powerful enough to bring benefits.

To use this strategy:

Ask your prescribing doctor about possible side effects. You can also consult a nurse or pharmacist. You may also want to check with both your doctor and your pharmacist to be sure that any new medication—including over-the-counter or nonprescription drugs—will not interact in harmful ways with what you're already taking.

You may also choose to read about your medications online or in reference books. But remember: those sources list every possible side effect, even rare ones. Don't let them alarm you unnecessarily.

Rely on the professionals who know you and your condition best. Use your Coping Notebook to record any side-effects that you experience—what happened, when it started, how long it lasted, and what you were taking. Contact your doctor or healthcare team about anything concerning, and seek urgent care for severe reactions (for example, trouble breathing, swelling of the face or throat, or fainting).

[ ] #81

Compartmentalize

Do you ever feel so overloaded with things to think about that you can't focus on anything? This is not unusual. But you want to do something about it.

You want to become more confident in your ability to separate what's less important from your true priorities. So even if there are a lot of overwhelming things going on, your goal is to compartmentalize—put the things you don't have to think about at the moment into an imaginary box. Then push it aside, so you can focus more intently on what is currently most important.

To use this strategy:

Try to organize the things on your mind and the things that need your attention. Divide them into different categories. Then imagine placing less urgent ones into separate compartments and setting them aside. Focus only on the compartment that matters most in the moment.

[ ] #82

Share the Responsibility of Decision-Making

There will inevitably be many decisions made as part of your treatment. But who is going to make those decisions? You? Your doctor? Anyone else?

You know yourself. Do you want to make all of your own decisions? It really is up to you, although you probably won't make all decisions without your treatment team's input. You'll want to get advice from professionals and significant others and use that advice to help your decision-making.

But what if you don't want to make all the decisions yourself? You don't have to. Decide who among your family, friends, and healthcare team you want to help make decisions for you, and speak to them about it.

To use this strategy:

In your Coping Notebook, write down your preferences for decision-making. When do you (appropriately!) want to be in charge? For what types of decisions? When would you prefer to lean on others? And for which decisions?

Ideally, you'll want to discuss, in advance, who will make decisions about what, and how to deal with disagreements with others who may share responsibility. This way no one (including you) has to carry the full weight of decision-making alone.

B- Strategies for Your Body and Symptoms

Every person with a chronic illness experiences symptoms, manifestations, and the course of their disease in their own way. Because each person is different, coping methods and adjustments must also be individualized.

That is why it's important to pay close attention to your own body and symptoms and determine how to live with your illness most effectively. Some strategies from earlier chapters can help, and the practical strategies in this section will give you additional tools.

[ ] #83

Focus on Your Body

The more you understand your body and how your illness affects it, the better off you are. In addition to being aware of what you're generally feeling physically, you want to become more tuned in to any factors that might trigger symptom onset or exacerbation. This will help you to feel more in control and limit any avoidable increase in symptoms.

Try to always be aware of what your body is telling you. You know your body better than anybody else. Your diagnosis means that you have more to learn and be aware of. Conversations with your doctor will help you understand what to watch for and when you may need to contact your doctor between visits.

To use this strategy:

Use the "Symptom Inventory" page of your Coping Notebook (see Strategy #18). Record when symptoms occur, to what degree, what triggers them, and how they change over time. Include any additional information that you (or your doctor) think is important. Look for patterns you can act on or report to your doctor.

[ ] #84

Store All Medical Information on Your Computer

As time goes by after your diagnosis, you're going to be accumulating a lot of information about your condition, including the doctors you see, your treatments, and your medications (including doses, ways in which you will take your pills, side effects, etc.). All of this is valuable information.

You want to include notes about all of this in your Coping Notebook, and there are a number of strategies in this book to help you to do that. But some people love computers. If that's you, it's also a good idea to keep all of your medical information on them. Like notebooks, computer files keep information accessible and organized, and they are easy to update.

Computers also make it easy to print out details for appointments or securely send information to healthcare providers (or others, as needed).

Keeping your information on the computer also helps if you have to go to a new doctor. You'll be able to print out any relevant information about your condition, and either send it in advance or bring it to your appointment. You won't have to try to explain your complete history over and over. This saves time and ensures accuracy.

To use this strategy:

Set up specific files on your computer for all of your medical information. Although you could keep all of your information in one file, it may make sense to set up different files for different aspects of your care (symptoms, treatments, medications, providers). Keep them updated and ready to print or share.

You'll want to include information from other parts of this book—such as your condition (see Strategy #20), your symptoms (see Strategy #18), your treatments (see Strategy #72), your medications (see Strategy #79), your treatment team (see Strategy #86), and anything else you may need to bring to current or new doctors. Linking these strategies together in one digital system will make your information easier to update and share.

[ ] #85

Be Prepared to Fill Out Online Questionnaires

In the age of electronic medical records, physicians often require new patients to fill out online questionnaires prior to their initial appointment. This may be a drudgery, but it's now standard practice. So be prepared for it

To use this strategy:

Have all relevant information at your fingertips (either in your Coping Notebook or in your computer file- See Strategy #84). This includes:

- Names and contact information for doctors (and other members of your healthcare team)
- Medication list, dosages, and start dates

- Symptom history
- Insurance details and ID numbers

See if you can print out a hard copy of any online questionnaires you have to fill out. This will help you to have the information available if you need to prepare future questionnaires (and will help you revise what you have in your Coping Notebook or on your computer) and will save you time later.

WHAT'S NEXT?

Everything you do to actively participate in your treatment makes you stronger and improves the way you work with your care team. In the next chapter, we'll look at how to put together the best treatment team possible and how to make the most of your interactions with health-care professionals.

I Need to Get the Right Care from the Right People

A big part of living well after diagnosis is learning how to work with the people who will guide your care. Your treatment team may include doctors, nurses, pharmacists, therapists, and mental health professionals—all playing different roles to help you. The more you take an active role in building and maintaining these relationships, the better your treatment and overall coping will be.

This chapter introduces strategies to help you put together your treatment team and work with them in a way that makes you an informed, active partner. Your goal is not just to follow instructions, but to take part in your care so you get the best possible help.

A- Dealing with Your Doctors

Living with a chronic illness rarely runs smoothly. Your doctors play a central role in your treatment, but the more prepared you are, the better you'll handle bumps along the way. A strong partnership with your doctor can make a big difference, helping you know what to watch for, when to call, and what you can do on your own to support your care.

The strategies in this section will help you get the most out of your working relationship with your doctors.

[ ] #86

Build Your Treatment Team

Who are the professionals who are going to be part of your treatment team? The size of your treatment team will vary, depending on your condition, its symptoms, and what treatment is necessary, among other factors.

Your entire treatment team doesn't have to be in place right away. It usually takes time for your team to come together, and sometimes new members are added if your needs change.

Your treatment team isn't limited to physicians. You can also include therapists, counselors, pharmacists, nurses, and other healthcare professionals who can help you manage your condition.

Each member of your treatment team should be aware of everyone else on your team, and any types of treatment that you are receiving, so that your care can be properly and efficiently coordinated.

Having all of this information in one place will help you get the most out of coordinated care.

To use this strategy:

Set up a section in your Coping Notebook for your treatment team. Then create a page for each professional involved in your care. Enter all contact information, including telephone numbers, e-mail addresses (if provided), mailing addresses, and specialties.

Leave space to jot down additional information, such as where you learned about the doctor, particular treatment recommendations, when to call and when not to call (more about this later), and other things you want to remember.

The first page in this section should be for the physician who will be your medical care coordinator. (See Strategy #88.) Add pages if/when new professionals join your team.

[ ] #87

Keep Key Contacts in One Place

It may seem obvious, but many people don't keep important contact information in one spot—and end up scrambling during stressful moments. When you're dealing with an illness, you don't want the extra burden of hunting for a phone number or e-mail address. Having everything in one place saves time and stress when you most need it.

To use this strategy:

Any address, phone number or e-mail address that may be important for you should be on one "Contact" page in your Coping Notebook. This should be in addition to, not instead of, where you normally keep numbers, like your phone or address book. Keeping a master list in your notebook ensures you always have a backup.

[ ] #88

Determine Who Your Medical Care Coordinator Is

Does your condition require you to see more than one doctor, possibly in different specialties? If this is the case, it's a good idea to have one primary doctor serve as your "go-to" person. This doctor will gather all information obtained from your different doctors and will be the "hub of the wheel" in helping you coordinate your different specialists.

Often, your main physician- the one who specializes in your condition-will fill this role. Other professionals may join your team, depending on your symptoms, your doctor's recommendations, and your medical and emotional needs.

To use this strategy:

Make sure that your medical care coordinator is comfortable with that role. If not, you may need to choose someone else with the necessary expertise and willingness to coordinate.

In your Coping Notebook, set up a page for the professional who will be your coordinator. Jot down what role they play, which other providers they need to stay in contact with, and any preferences or instructions they've given you. This gives you a clear picture of who is overseeing your care, helps keep your team coordinated, and makes it easy to update information as things change.

[ ] #89

Maintain a Good Working Relationship with Your Doctors

The teamwork approach between patient and doctor is critical to the success of your care. Your doctor will bring medical experience and insight to your treatment. You'll bring (hopefully) a willingness to play an active role in your treatment, as well as to follow treatment plans.

There are so many reasons to have a good relationship with your doctors. For example, you'll get the best possible care, you'll foster feelings of mutual respect ... and your calls will most likely be taken when you need to get information or report symptoms!

But what if this is occasionally more difficult than you expected? What if you're frustrated, not feeling well, or have difficulty reaching your doctor?

The most important component in any relationship (with anyone) is communication. You need to feel comfortable enough with each member of your treatment team to bring up questions or concerns when needed. You need to trust them, listen to them, follow their advice, and question them when you're unsure. This is all part of a good partnership…such an important goal in your healthcare.

To use this strategy:

In your Coping Notebook, set up a page to jot down any issues of discomfort that you're having with any of your doctors. This doesn't mean you should go looking for problems—but it does mean you shouldn't ignore issues that bother you.

Then jot down your plan for what you're going to do about this, as well as a clear goal for resolving this discomfort. How are you going to approach the professional? What are you going to say? If you're really uncomfortable, you may even want to "script" what you want to say, to make sure it comes out as calmly and constructively as possible.

If any issues of discomfort are critical, act on them right away. If not, just keep track of them until your next appointment with this doctor, when you can bring it up directly. (If you're uncomfortable with how to do that, talk to members of your support team- see Chapter 7- about how to broach a potentially uncomfortable conversation.)

[ ] #90

Avoid, or Modify, Expectations

Early on, following the diagnosis of a medical condition, you may want to gather every bit of information you can, or you may feel so overwhelmed that you'd rather not think about your condition at all. Either way, it's common to hope your doctor will figure everything out right away. But it's important to keep your expectations realistic.

Your doctor is trying to help, and won't turn away from what you're going through, delay treatment unnecessarily, or avoid finding out helpful information. However, there may be times when test results or treatment decisions take longer than you would like.

Work with your doctor. Discuss the schedule and process for getting as much information as possible, and learn about the timetable for your treatment. Anticipate those times when delays frustrate you, and remind yourself that waiting is sometimes part of the process. Try to avoid having unrealistic expectations. (See Strategy #112 for more about expectations.)

To use this strategy:

In your Coping Notebook, create a double-column page for your expectations. On the left side, write down the expectations you have about your doctor, your treatment, or your progress (for example, *"I expect my doctor to have all the answers right away"* or *"I expect my treatment to work without side effects"*). On the right side, write a more realistic version of each expectation (for example, *"My doctor may need time to get test results before deciding on the next step"* or *"Most treatments help, but side effects are sometimes part of the process"*).

By comparing both sides, you'll see where your expectations may need adjusting. This exercise can reduce frustration, remind you of what's realistic, and help you stay more patient with yourself and your treatment team.

[ ] #91

Know When to Call Your Doctor

Because it's so important to have a good relationship with your doctor, you want to know when to call (and when not to call) to ask questions or report symptoms.

You may be concerned that calling too often will make you appear to be a pest. On the other hand, if you don't call when you should, you may not be reporting important information that your doctor needs to guide your care.

All doctors have preferences as to when patients should call them. It's important for you to know each doctor's preferences.

Are there particular symptoms that need to be reported? Side effects from medications? Questions about the condition itself? What to do when ...? These are just some of the things that you'll want to know. How do you find out? They'll often tell you. Otherwise, just ask!

To use this strategy:

Use your Coping Notebook to keep all of this information in one place. As discussed in Strategy #86, you'll have a separate page for each doctor. Add this information to your doctor's page as you learn more about your doctor's preferences. Then you'll be able to refer to this information in the future, when you may find yourself wondering, "Should I call, or shouldn't I?"

You'll also be writing down all information about your symptoms. (See Strategy #18.) You'll be accumulating information that you may want to share with your doctor. You'll learn which information you can discuss at your next scheduled appointment, or which you need to bring to your doctor's attention right away.

You also want to know how to get in touch with your doctor. More and more doctors are providing e-mail addresses for questions. In addition, many offices now use secure patient portals where you can send messages, review results, and ask non-urgent questions. If the phone is the only form of contact, you'll want to know when your doctor is available, when the doctor would prefer you to call, and what to do if you need to call outside of normal office hours. This also should be on each doctor's individual page.

[ ] #92

Consult Your Doctor Before Considering Any Treatment Changes

There may be times when, for some reason, you believe changes should be made in your treatment. For example, you may have read something about your condition, heard comments at a support group, or felt that your treatment just wasn't working. You may be experiencing a difference in your symptoms, a new side effect to your medication, or are not responding to treatment the way you did before.

Please remember this: it's not a good idea to make changes, especially significant ones, on your own. Make sure you discuss any thoughts you have about changes with your doctor. This is true even if the changes you're considering are not medical (e.g., adding exercise, using other treatment modalities, introducing nutritional supplements).

After all, your doctor is your treatment partner; you should be able to discuss these things without hesitation. If you feel that you can't bring anything up with your doctor, try first to bring this up directly. If you still feel uncomfortable, it may be a sign that your doctor-patient relationship is not as open or supportive as it should be.

[ ] #93

Give... and Receive... Respect

One of the most important components of a healthy relationship with your doctors and other support professionals is mutual respect. Not only is it important for you to respect the person you're working with, but it's important for you to feel respected back.

Remember that your doctor is a person first. Speak to your doctor as you would want to be spoken to, and don't be afraid to speak up when something matters to you.

It is important that you be able to communicate with your doctors about your condition, its treatment, and your "partnership." If you can't communicate with your doctor, what kind of partnership do you truly have?

Good doctors want to know what you're thinking, and what's troubling you, not just about your symptoms. If there is something that's bothering you, it's important to discuss this. However, treat your doctor with the respect that you'd want in return. If you come on too strong, you may unintentionally strain the relationship and make it harder to work together productively.

If you're not able to communicate with your doctor, resentment may build up inside of you, and this can affect you psychologically, as well as interfere with your treatment itself.

This doesn't mean that you should call your doctor every time something bothers you. (You may still need to set up a consultation appointment for your doctor's time.) Remember, your goal is to do what you can to maintain the quality of your partnership.

Treat your doctor with courtesy. Be honest and share information willingly and appropriately. Establish trust from the get-go. Communicate about any concerns that may arise in the relationship. Aim to truly work together as teammates. Hopefully, you'll receive all of these back from your doctor as well.

To use this strategy:

In your Coping Notebook, turn to the page for each of the professionals who are currently part of your team. Then jot down the answers to the following questions:

- What kind of relationship do you currently have?
- Do you respect them?
- Do you feel they respect you?
- For those needing improvement, what can you do to improve this?
- How are you going to do this?

Then keep track of your progress in building mutual respect.

[ ] #94

Know When and Why to Go for a Second Opinion

At one time or another, virtually everyone living with a chronic illness goes for a second opinion. This may especially be useful following your diagnosis in order to confirm it. After all, you want to have the best and most accurate foundation to move forward.

It is common to feel confused following the diagnosis of a chronic illness. This is particularly true if you've been blindsided by a diagnosis you weren't expecting at all.

The questions that pop into your mind may often include: Is the diagnosis correct? What am I supposed to do now? Are the recommended treatments truly the best treatments for my condition?

These and other questions make it reasonable to consider going for a second opinion. The more serious or potentially life-threatening your newly diagnosed condition is, the more important this can be.

In addition, a second opinion will help you learn even more about the diagnosis and your condition. The more knowledgeable you are, the better. It will help you make more accurate, informed decisions about your recommended treatment. You'll be able to ask additional questions that may come to mind, even the same questions, to see if the answers match the answers you've already received.

You'll be able to discuss alternatives to your current treatment plan. You'll also find out what outcomes and prognoses are anticipated by the second opinion doctor. You'll be able to compare all of this information to what your first doctor told you.

However, you're not obligated to do this. If you are confident in the doctor who diagnosed you, and the methodology used, as well as everything you've learned thus far, you may choose not to go for a second opinion. In some cases, you may not want to think about it anymore, or don't want go through another series of tests or appointments. (Although, is that truly a good reason not to consider a second opinion?)

Finally, remember that a second opinion isn't always right. You want to make sure that your diagnosis is correct. You may not be happy if the second opinion confirms the initial diagnosis, but at least you can be more secure in that diagnosis. On the other hand, if there's disagreement, that signals the need for more exploration into what's going on.

Regardless of what happens with your second opinion, be aware of (and try to avoid) "doctor-shopping" ... going for more and more opinions, looking for someone who will tell you what you *want* to hear.

To use this strategy:

Before you even broach the idea of a second opinion to your doctor, write down the answers to the following questions:

- Why am I looking to go for a second opinion?
- What questions do I want answered when I go?
- What will I do if the answers are different from what I've already been told?

Your written responses will help you organize your thoughts and prepare for the second opinion appointment.

[ ] #95

Know What to Say When Mentioning a Second Opinion

Often, one of the hardest things for patients is to mention the idea of a second opinion to their doctor. Some people even hesitate about getting other opinions because they're afraid of offending their doctor or seeming not to believe them.

Good doctors know better. They almost always are receptive to the idea of a second opinion. And, remember: the same way that you may be looking to go for a second opinion to another doctor, there will likely be people who come to your current doctor for second opinions as well.

If you are nervous about bringing this up, remember that honesty with your doctor is crucial. Most good doctors will be supportive of you getting another opinion. If it validates their own, at least you'll all know that there is agreement about the diagnosis and its implications. On the other hand, if there is any disagreement, good doctors will want to understand the reasons for this, so it can be best determined how to proceed.

You'll feel more comfortable when your doctor agrees to your getting a second opinion. (If you encounter resistance, however, ask yourself why—they may be uncomfortable for reasons worth exploring.)

No matter how uncomfortable you might feel about this, don't go behind your doctor's back. You'll need your records, charts, or test results for that second opinion anyway, so somehow your doctor will likely find out. And, of course, you'll want your second opinion doctor to be able to consult with your original doctor as needed.

To use this strategy:

Before you bring up the idea of a second opinion to your doctor, remind yourself of why you want it, and prepare a calm way to say it. Practice a simple, respectful phrase you can use. For example:

- "I'm so overwhelmed by all of this. It may help me to hear another opinion, just so I know I'm moving forward with confidence."

Be positive, friendly, and polite when you raise the subject. Frame it as wanting the most accurate information to move forward, not as doubting your doctor.

Remember, many good doctors even suggest second opinions themselves. If your doctor encourages it, don't assume they lack confidence in your case—see it as a sign of professionalism and teamwork.

[ ] #96
Know Who to Go to for a Second Opinion

If and when you go for a second opinion, who should you see?

It is often strongly recommended that you go to somebody who is not connected with your primary doctor. Why? If it's important enough to get another opinion, it's important that it be an independent second opinion. Any consultation between them should take place *after* the second opinion, rather than beforehand.

You want the specialty of your second opinion doctor to be the same as your primary treating doctor's specialty, unless you're going for an opinion about a symptom that might benefit from a different specialty.

One of the concerns that people have about second opinions is that it's going to cost them more money. Many insurance companies willingly cover second opinions, figuring that getting the correct diagnosis and treatment recommendations will ultimately save them money. If there is any hesitancy on the part of your insurance company, discuss this with your current doctor.

One final thought: If you find that you're uncomfortable with your current doctor, going for a second opinion can be a good way to learn about other doctors who treat your condition.

In this modern age, there are even legitimate online services that can provide second opinions in some cases. If this is something you'd consider, make sure to only contact a reputable organization, such as the Cleveland Clinic, New York Presbyterian, or Johns Hopkins.

Here's a tip: Many leading hospitals post helpful guides about second opinions online. Even if you don't use their services, browsing these resources can give you a clearer idea of what to expect and what to prepare.

To use this strategy:

Start planning who you might see for a second opinion. Ask both professionals and people in your support network for leads to trustworthy doctors.

In your Coping Notebook, continue adding to your list of questions, using the double-column method to track both questions and answers.

Make sure you write down everything you learn at the second opinion visit so you can compare it with what your current doctor has told you.

[ ] #97

Know When to Stay, and If/When to Leave Your Doctor

As we've discussed before, the need for a good working partnership with your doctor is critical. There may be times, though, that you may feel that the relationship with your doctor just isn't working. Unless you feel very strongly about this, it's a good idea to have a conversation with your doctor before making any change.

Remember, you're not obligated to stay with any doctor who makes you uncomfortable. This is not advocating doctor-shopping or jumping around from person to person until you get the diagnosis or treatment regimen that you really want. Instead, it's important to be mindful about whether the relationship with your doctor is working or not.

To use this strategy:

In your Coping Notebook, set up a page to help you decide whether or not you are going to proceed in changing doctors. Then answer the following questions:

- What am I hoping to accomplish by changing?
- How am I going to discuss this with the doctor?
- What was the outcome of any discussions?

This will help you to make a practical decision about what you're going to do.

[ ] #98

Don't Avoid Your Doctors

There are some people who feel that they're bothering their doctors. They may fear that they're going too often and, as such, will become an annoyance. So, they may avoid or delay appointments, sometimes for extended periods of time. Is this truly in your best interest? The more time that goes by, the more your doctor has to catch up on with you and your condition.

Your doctors will tell you how often they want to see you. Adhere to that frequency. Don't feel that you're doing yourself or your doctor a favor by not going as often, or seeing how long you can stretch out the time between visits.

What if your doctor does not set a specific next appointment for you? They may suggest that you let them know when you need to make an appointment. Ask if any symptoms or instructions would necessitate calling for an appointment.

Keep a list of anything noteworthy that occurs between appointments. Don't let the list become lengthy. When there are significant items on that list, it's time to call the doctor for an appointment. You don't have to be in crisis to make an appointment.

To use this strategy:

Use your Coping Notebook to jot down any symptoms, side effects, or concerns as they occur. When the list reaches a point where it feels important or is affecting your daily life, schedule an appointment—even if you're not in crisis. This ensures problems are addressed before they grow larger.

[ ] #99

Develop a Good Relationship with Your Doctor's Support Staff

The best way to get through to your doctor is to have a supportive staff member recognize when there is a need to connect. The friendlier you are to the support staff, the more likely they are to "be on your side." And, as they get to know you, they'll recognize that you only call when you really need to. (Make sure that's true!)

To use this strategy:

Make a list of the names of the support staff in your doctors' offices. As you get to know them, jot down details that may help you remember who's who and what they do.

When you call, smile *before* you speak. Let them hear warmth in your voice. Always express your appreciation for what they do. Remember, courtesy goes a long way toward building a supportive connection.

B- Dealing with Your Medical Appointments

The most important interaction you have with the members of your medical team is often at appointments. This is the one place where you can count on their undivided attention, learn the latest information, and ask your questions. It makes sense, therefore, to do everything you can to prepare in order to maximize their benefits.

In this section, you'll find strategies to help you get the most out of every visit. You'll learn how to set goals for your appointments, prepare notes in advance, prioritize your questions, and even handle newer formats like telehealth. The better prepared you are, the more useful and productive each appointment will be.

[ ] #100

Know Your Purpose for Each Appointment

Are you going for an appointment because it is a routine, scheduled part of your treatment, because something has come up and you need to be checked out, or for some other reason? This will determine the amount and type of preparation you'll want to do.

When you set up an appointment, ask yourself: What's my goal? Is it to adjust treatment, get my doctor's opinion on progress, confirm next steps, seek reassurance, or talk through emotions connected to my condition?

The more you know about why you've scheduled your appointment, the better you can prepare and benefit from it.

To use this strategy:

In your Coping Notebook, write down the specific reason for each appointment. Is it for treatment, information, reassurance, or problem-solving? This will help you focus, stay on track during the visit, and measure whether your goal was met. Make sure to remember to write notes either during or following your appointment.

[ ] #101
Prepare for Each Appointment in Advance

Before any doctor's appointment, put together all current, relevant information about your symptoms and treatment.

To use this strategy:

Jot down everything you want to discuss at your next appointment, so you won't forget important details. Include:

- What current symptoms you're experiencing (the specific symptom, frequency, intensity, duration)

- What treatments you're receiving (including medication dosage, how it helps, side effects)
- Any other consultations, treatments, lab work, or scans since your last visit (and whether results were sent to your doctor)
- Any new symptoms—describe what they feel like, when they started, how long they last, and what makes them better or worse.

You may find it useful to rate symptom intensity on a 0–10 scale (0 = none, 10 = worst imaginable).

Also prepare information about how your treatment is going overall. What's working well? What difficulties are you experiencing, and when do they occur?

Having this written out means you'll walk in with confidence, ready to get the most out of your time.

[ ] #102

Prepare for Telehealth Visits

Telehealth can save time and make care more accessible. But just like in-person visits, preparation matters. If you're scrambling with tech problems, searching for your medication bottles, or distracted by background noise, you lose valuable minutes of your appointment. Treat a telehealth visit as seriously as an office appointment: show up prepared, minimize distractions, and keep your notes close at hand.

To use this strategy:

Before your telehealth visit, test your camera, microphone, and internet connection. Make sure your device is charged or plugged in. Choose a quiet, well-lit spot where you'll have privacy, and let others know not to disturb you. Have your Coping Notebook open to your symptom notes, your question list, and your treatment information. Keep your medications and recent results nearby in case your doctor asks. Finally, ask the office how to follow up if questions come up after the call—through the patient portal, by phone, or by email.

[ ] #103

Prioritize Your Questions for Each Appointment

It is an unfortunate fact in today's medical world that you only have a certain amount of time with your doctor at each appointment. Therefore, it's important to organize and prioritize what you want to talk about during your appointment. That means deciding which symptoms to report, which questions to ask first, and which concerns can wait.

To use this strategy:

In Strategy #19, we talked about setting up a question-and-answer page. You'll use that page often throughout your care. For each appointment, create a new page dedicated to that visit.

Try to limit the number of priority questions you plan on asking. More than that may take too much time. You can write down lower-priority questions lower on the page, just in case you zip through your priority questions. (We'll discuss shortly what to do about questions that you're not able to get answered at your appointment.)

Here are examples of questions you might ask. What do my symptoms mean? What can I do about them? Are there additional treatments or lifestyle steps I should take? What should I do if things get worse? How will treatment affect my daily life? What should I avoid? Who do I contact with questions after hours?

Obviously, you can add to this list if there are important questions that you've noted since your last visit.

Make sure to leave space to write answers as you go. Keep track of lower priority questions that you did not ask. They may be useful for your next visit.

[ ] #104

Report Symptoms, but Get Feedback

Here's something that frustrates many patients: They go to medical appointments, report their symptoms, the doctor diligently records them... but then there's no feedback. If you don't know what your symptoms mean, whether to worry, or what steps to take, you can leave more anxious than when you arrived. Reporting symptoms is important, but it's only part of the job—you also need to ask what those symptoms suggest and what to do about them.

To use this strategy:

If you're concerned about what symptoms mean, ask in the moment. Simple questions like, "What does it mean when I feel _______?" or, "What should I do if this happens again?" make your reporting more useful.

In your Coping Notebook, prepare a page for symptoms that concern you. List the symptoms and leave space to record your doctor's response. This way you not only report your symptoms, you also leave with clear guidance on what they mean and what to do.

[ ] #105

Take Notes, but Keep Listening

It's natural to want to capture everything your doctor says, but writing too much can actually make you miss important information. Stress and worry can also cloud your memory, making it harder to recall details later. If you try to write down everything that your doctor is saying, you may find that you miss some of the information you need to hear.

A simple system for note-taking helps you keep the essentials without losing focus in the moment.

To use this strategy:

During appointments, try to jot down key words or phrases only, something that will jog your memory later. Flesh them out right after the appointment while the details are still fresh. If something is especially important, don't hesitate to ask your doctor to repeat it. That way, you can keep listening while still capturing what matters most.

[ ] #106
Bring Extra Ears

Appointments can be overwhelming. You may be trying to absorb new information, keep track of symptoms, and remember your own questions—all while managing stress. That's why many patients leave appointments realizing they've missed something important. Bringing someone you trust gives you backup, reassurance, and an extra set of ears to catch what you might overlook.

To use this strategy:

Ask a supportive friend or family member to join you when possible. Their role is to listen, take notes, and remind you of your questions if you get sidetracked. In your Coping Notebook, make a page for potential helpers and jot down their availability and strengths. Be practical; consider the person's age, ability to handle responsibility, and comfort in medical settings.

Before each appointment, explain what you need from them—mainly to listen and help recall answers afterward. After the visit, compare notes so you leave with a fuller, more accurate record of what was said. If no one is available to come with you, ask your doctor's office whether you can record the visit (with permission) or plan extra time afterward to write down everything while it's still fresh.

[ ] #107
Write Down What You've Learned as Soon as Possible

Even if you've taken notes during your appointment—or brought someone with you—it's easy to forget details once you leave. Stress, information overload, and the rush to get back to your day all chip away at memory. The sooner you record what you've learned, the more accurate and complete your notes will be. Small details that seem obvious in the moment can fade quickly if you wait too long.

To use this strategy:

After your appointment, take a few minutes to write down everything you remember while it's still fresh. If possible, sit in the waiting room or your car before leaving and review your notes. Add details, fill in gaps, and highlight anything you want to follow up on. If someone comes with you, compare notes so you can build a clearer picture together.

Keep these notes in your Coping Notebook, either on your Question/Answer page or on a dedicated page for each appointment. This way, when you look back, you'll have a reliable record of what was said, what steps to take, and what you may want to ask at your next visit.

[ ] #108

Determine What to Do with Additional Questions or Confusion

It's rare to leave an appointment with every answer clear and no questions left. You may not understand everything you were told, or you may later realize something was missing. If that happens, it's important to know what to do.

The first thing to do is to determine if your question or concern is urgent. If it can wait, write it on your question/answer page for your next appointment. If it can't, you'll want to follow up sooner. Knowing when and how to follow up helps you feel more comfortable reaching out without worrying about being a nuisance.

To use this strategy:

Write your questions or areas of confusion in your Coping Notebook right after the appointment. If the matter is urgent, call your doctor's office. If not, ask a staff member how best to send non-urgent questions—many doctors prefer you use their patient portal.

You can also clarify this directly with your doctor: ask, "If I have questions between visits, what's the best way to reach you?" Having that answer in advance helps you feel confident about following up.

C- Dealing with Mental Health Professionals

Physicians aren't the only healthcare professionals who may be part of your treatment team. Nurses, therapists, counselors, and others can all play important roles in supporting your care.

Because your diagnosis affects both your body and your mind, a mental health professional may be an important member of your team. This section introduces strategies for finding the right professional, feeling comfortable with your choice, and making the most of your sessions.

[ ] #109

Include Support Professionals on Your Team

There may be times following your diagnosis (and during your life with your condition), when you feel overwhelmed or unable to cope. That's when it's important not to hesitate to reach out to trained professionals who can help. Working with a mental health professional can give you strategies to better manage the emotional side of your illness.

So, who do you go to if you decide you'd like extra support? There are many types of mental health professionals who can help, including psychiatrists, psychologists, social workers, and counselors. Not all may have experience with chronic illness, but many do, and they can be valuable resources.

There are also many ways to find them:

- Ask your doctors first. They regularly see patients who need this kind of support and usually know trusted professionals to recommend.
- Talk to nurses or physician assistants in your doctor's office.
- Call a local chapter of a health organization related to your condition.
- Ask people in a support group or others living with your illness. Word-of-mouth referrals are often especially valuable.
- Even your pharmacist may have heard of professionals through conversations with other patients.
- Contact local chapters of professional associations, such as medical societies or psychological associations.

- Libraries, hospitals, and reputable online directories can also provide leads.

The more you network, the more likely you'll find someone who feels like a good fit.

To use this strategy:

In your Coping Notebook, create a page for potential mental health professionals. Write down names and contact information from any leads you gather. As you make calls or check referrals, jot down what you learn—such as their specialty, experience with your condition, and availability. Later, you can use this information to compare options and decide who might best support you.

[ ] #110
Feel Comfortable Selecting a Mental Health Professional

There are many professionals in the mental health field, but not every one will be the right fit for you. A good match matters because comfort and trust are key to progress. Asking a few questions at the beginning can help you decide if someone is right for you.

To use this strategy:

In your Coping Notebook, create a page for each professional you contact. Write down answers to questions such as:

- Do you have experience working with people who have my condition?
- What kinds of approaches or therapies do you use?
- How often would we meet, and for how long?
- What are your fees, and do you accept my insurance?

Your notes will help you compare and decide whether you feel comfortable moving forward.

[ ] #111

Keep Track of Issues to Discuss with Your Mental Health Professional

What are your goals in talking with a mental health professional? The more you know what you're trying to accomplish, the more benefit you will derive. These goals may change over time, so keeping track of them is important.

To use this strategy:

Use a small notebook or a section of your Coping Notebook specifically for mental health sessions. Write down issues, questions, or concerns as they come up in your daily life. Examples might include:

- How to talk with your kids if you're too tired to spend time with them
- What to say to your boss about your diagnosis
- How to manage fear before medical appointments
- Coping with frustration when progress feels slow

Bring your notebook to each session. Jot down your therapist's answers and suggestions so you can review them later and track your progress.

WHAT'S NEXT?

This chapter focused on working with your treatment team—from doctors and staff to mental health professionals. By building partnerships, asking questions, and preparing for each appointment, you take an active role in your care. The next chapter turns inward, focusing on strengthening your inner self. You'll learn strategies to support your mental health, build emotional strength, and find balance as you continue your journey.

CHAPTER 7

I Need to Strengthen My Mindset and Resilience

You are not simply a patient—you are a whole person. The stronger you are on the inside, emotionally and mentally, the more effectively you can cope with illness and living well after diagnosis.

This chapter introduces strategies to strengthen your inner self. Some may feel more useful to you than others. Experiment and adopt those that best support your journey.

A- Support Yourself with Healthy Thinking

Your goal is not to be defined by your illness. Your goal is to fit your illness into who you are. One of the best ways to do this is to work on your thinking.

The way you think can be your best friend ... or your worst enemy.

Make it your friend by catching yourself when negative thoughts or emotions creep in. Often, it's not the situation itself that brings you down, but the way you think about it.

Turning negative thoughts into realistic, happier ones will help to strengthen your inner self.

[ ] #112

Try to Have Realistic Expectations

The word "expectation" is a dangerous word. If you expect something a certain way, you open yourself up to the risk of being emotionally devastated if it doesn't turn out that way. So, if you have expectations (for example, of yourself, your doctors, or your treatment), you can become very upset if things don't turn out the way you anticipated.

Try to be realistic in the way you approach everything about your condition. No pill is going to make your chronic illness go away. No professional is going to have the perfect treatment plan. No family member or friend is going to be there for you 100% of the time. It's not going to be sunny every day.

Regardless of what's going on with your health following your diagnosis, there is always room for something positive to happen. Learning to take the inevitable ups and downs in stride will help you to cope better.

To use this strategy:

Work on changing your thinking when you catch yourself expecting something. (For example, "I expect that my blood work will be normal at my next doctor's visit." Or, "I expect that I'll be able to get to my daughter's meeting at school.")

Change your "expect" thoughts to "it would be nice" thoughts. (For example, "I hope that my blood work will be normal, but I'll deal with it if it isn't." Or, "I hope to get to my daughter's meeting at school, but she loves me and will be OK if I can't.") Changing your language softens the thought, making you less vulnerable to emotional swings.

If you find that a lot of your thinking involves expectations, you may want to use the double-column technique in your Coping Notebook. Write down your "expect" thought on the left side of the page, and then rewrite it using "it would be nice" language (or something similar) on the right side.

[ ] #113

Be Nice to Yourself

The nicer you are to yourself, the more you can adjust your condition. So, how do you do that?

People can adapt, even to the most difficult of circumstances. Keep reminding yourself of that. There is every reason to believe that you will be able to learn to move forward following your diagnosis. Give that a chance to happen, even if there are times when it feels impossible. No pressure.

There are times when it will be harder than others. You may be more upset with yourself at some times than at others. Focus on being understanding, compassionate, and supportive of yourself, even then. Would you be nice to others if you saw them going through a hard time? Of course, you would. So, be the same way to yourself.

Support yourself. Keep telling yourself, "I can do this! I can do this! I am strong!" Wouldn't you tell this to a loved one to motivate them if they were in your position? Then why not tell yourself the same thing?

As each day passes, whether you've gone for a treatment, another doctor's appointment, or have even done something important that you had to accomplish that day, think about how strong you are to have met that challenge. Keep thinking this way to feel better about yourself.

Make sure your mood and attitude are as positive as possible. We all talk to ourselves. You want to make sure that the way you talk to yourself is as gentle, supportive, and encouraging as it can be. Reassure yourself that you will feel more like yourself again as you learn how to fit your illness into your new normal.

What seems confusing at first will eventually start to make sense. These may be some of the biggest changes you've ever faced. Give yourself time to adjust. You can learn how to take care of yourself and your illness.

To use this strategy:

If you find that you're having difficulty doing this, be more aggressive in your efforts. (It's that important!) Set up a page in your Coping Notebook specifically for writing nice, self-supporting comments that you can say to yourself. Anytime you think or do something positive, write it down. It will feel good when you write it in the first place. And it will help you when you're down by being able to read things that you've written previously.

[ ] #114
Practice Self-Compassion

Many people living with illness are tougher on themselves than anyone else would be. Maybe you've thought, "I should be stronger," or "I'm letting people down." That inner voice drains the energy you need for coping.

Self-compassion means talking to yourself the way you would talk to someone you love who's going through the same thing—with patience, warmth, and perspective. It's not about ignoring problems, but about treating yourself with kindness while you face them.

To use this strategy:

The goal of this strategy is to shift from self-criticism to self-kindness. When you notice your inner critic speaking up, pause and take a slow breath. Gently ask yourself, "Would I say this to a friend?" If the answer is no, translate the thought into kinder, more accurate language to say to yourself. It can help to keep a ready phrase for tough moments—something like, "This is hard, and I'm doing my best." (You'll find more ideas for supportive phrases in Strategy #123.) Practicing this strategy will strengthen the habit so you'll naturally be kinder to yourself.

[ ] #115
Rebuild Your Self-Esteem and Self-Confidence

Self-esteem refers to the way you feel about yourself. Self-confidence refers to how you feel about the things that you do. These are similar concepts, but not exactly the same.

Has the way you feel about yourself been damaged because of your diagnosis? Research has shown that people may be so unhappy about being diagnosed with an illness that they feel worse about themselves. That's a double blow. Having your self-esteem damaged by your diagnosis can interfere with your attempts to move forward in a positive way.

You may not like yourself as much as you did before you were diagnosed. You may find yourself questioning whether you have the confidence to cope with any significant changes brought on by your diagnosis. These and other doubting questions are normal and understandable, but you don't want to give into these doubts. There's a lot that you can do to feel better about yourself.

Nurture your self-esteem. Keep focusing on the good things about you, the things you liked about yourself before you were diagnosed (and can still like after your diagnosis!). Remind yourself of all the things you've been able to accomplish in your life. Even if you're not able to be exactly the way you were before the diagnosis, this was not your doing. Therefore, you shouldn't feel worse about yourself.

Keep the whole experience of your diagnosis as one component of your life, not your whole life. Don't let it overshadow everything else.

To use this strategy:

Say nice things to yourself. The key to building and maintaining your self-esteem and self-confidence is the consistency with which you say positive messages to yourself. Make sure you keep this up, and don't let self-doubts or worries about your future with illness tear you down.

This needs to be an ongoing, conscious activity. Negative thoughts affecting your self-esteem can creep into your mind at any time, even on a subconscious level. Keep pumping yourself up. Keep focusing on your strengths. And make your commitment to working on bouncing back from your diagnosis a central part of feeling good about yourself.

[ ] #116
Focus on Your Body's Strengths

A lot of your thinking probably focuses on your symptoms, and how they make you feel worse about your body. Unfortunately, this is common. When people have medical problems, they tend to spend too much time lamenting how their bodies are not working properly.

Here's something you can do to help yourself: Try to focus on how parts of your body continue to function well. Thinking about the positives can help you balance out some of the negatives happening to your body.

To use this strategy:

Think about each part of your body, from your head to your toes. In your Coping Notebook, list the ways each body part continues to function well. Add to this list as you can. Refer to this information as a positive reminder whenever you slip into feeling that your body is letting you down.

[ ] #117

Don't Beat Yourself Up

Have you thought (or even had people say) that you brought your diagnosis on yourself? Has it been implied that you wouldn't have been diagnosed with your condition if you had taken better care of yourself, eaten better, exercised more, or reduced stress? How insulting!

Regardless of what anyone might inappropriately say, or even what you might think from time to time, there is no point in blaming yourself for the onset of your chronic illness. What do you really accomplish by doing this? Is this a way to help yourself? It won't help you, it won't change your diagnosis, and it won't make you better. Stay away from this type of negative thinking.

Instead, go into coping mode. Focus your thoughts on asking yourself: "I've been diagnosed, now what am I going to do about it? What am I going to do to help myself to move forward?" Isn't that a better way to think? Use your mental energy to help yourself, not beat on yourself.

[ ] #118

Give Yourself Permission Not to Think

Many of the strategies described in this book focus on different things that you can and should do to change your thinking. They are all valuable, but sometimes, enough is enough.

There are times when it is perfectly fine for you to give yourself permission not to think. Telling yourself that, however, may be as effective as telling yourself not to breathe!

So, if you think there are times when you want a break from thinking about your illness, make sure that you are prepared with other ways to redirect your mental energy.

Have distraction strategies available: things to do, things to read, positive things to say to yourself, or anything similar that will focus your attention elsewhere. You could even use a "thought-stopping" strategy, such as snapping your wrist with a rubber band, to keep yourself focused on something other than your thinking. (See also Strategy #8, in Chapter 1, or Strategy #59, in Chapter 3.)

B- Aim for a Positive Mental Attitude

Professional athletes don't tell themselves, "I can't do it". They tell themselves not only that they can do it, but that they will do it. So, they have the right attitude.

As you deal with your diagnosis, your mental attitude is more important than ever. This section discusses the importance of being positive, and how this can help you to achieve your goals in dealing with your illness.

[ ] #119

Think Positively

With everything that you're going through following your diagnosis, you may have a harder time thinking positively. But this is something you may need to remind yourself to do, over and over.

It's easy to get caught up in negativity at stressful times. However, the more you can consciously remind yourself to think positively, the more you can help yourself cope with your diagnosis, manage stress, and push back against negativity.

This may sound easier said than done. However, it is a goal that you can work on improving. So, stay focused. Catch those times when your thinking is slipping into "negative" territory, and rescue yourself by turning your thinking around in a positive direction.

To use this strategy:

If this is hard for you, use your double-column strategy and, on the left side, write the negative thoughts that automatically pop into your mind. Then on the right side, rewrite them in a more positive, realistic way. If you have difficulty rewriting any negatives, ask yourself what someone you respect would say if they had that negative thought, or what you would say to a friend or family member if they expressed that same thought to you.

This is similar to the rewriting technique, called cognitive restructuring, that we first discussed in Strategy #14. If you continue to have difficulty with this, talking to a mental health professional may help you to get your thinking to move in a more positive, helpful direction.

[ ] #120
Practice Mindfulness Meditation

Mindfulness reduces anxiety and helps you stay present, rather than getting pulled into fears about the future or regrets about the past.

Your mind may try to live in yesterday ("Why did this happen?") or tomorrow ("What if it gets worse?"). Mindfulness gently brings you back to now—the only place you can breathe, choose, and act. You don't need special equipment; even a few minutes can help.

To use this strategy:

Start small and be consistent. Sit comfortably and focus your attention on your breathing— air going in, air going out. When your mind wanders (and it will), notice this without judgment and gently return to your breath. If it helps, try a brief guided practice to get started. Over time, add a minute or two to your meditation as it feels right.

There are many good books and apps that can support your practice. Take advantage of whatever makes it easier to show up regularly.

[ ] #121
Build and Strengthen a Positive Mental Attitude

If you ask people who are handling their diagnoses well how they do it, you'll invariably find that one of the keys to their success is their positive mental attitude.

The more positive you are, the more you are able to help yourself. People who are more positive also tend to be more proactive, eat better, sleep more, engage more in treatment, feel more optimistic about the future, interact better with family, and more.

On the other hand, having a negative mental attitude can sabotage your treatment efforts. Research has shown that a negative outlook can adversely affect your immune system. It can also exacerbate feelings of anxiety and depression, which can adversely affect your body and your treatment. So, having a positive outlook can improve your life, your body, and the results of treatment.

It may be tough to have a positive mental attitude following your diagnosis. So be realistic. Even if your attitude takes a hit, this is something to work on. Don't just give in to it. Work to make your attitude more positive.

But what if you fear that you'll never have a positive attitude since you now have a chronic illness? Nonsense! Anyone can learn to improve their attitude. You can too! It involves working on your thinking (sound familiar?), identifying thoughts that reflect a negative mental attitude, and learning to turn them around.

For example, try to keep focusing on your glass as being half full instead of half empty. Instead of saying, "I'm doomed now that I've been diagnosed," say "OK, I now know what I have to deal with. Let's see what I can do about it."

As you try to keep your attitude positive, it is inevitable that some negative thoughts will sneak in there. Be ready for them. Be committed to pushing away these negative thoughts and replacing them with more realistic positive ones. Yes, this takes effort, especially when you're not feeling as good as you'd like to feel. The more you work on this, the more successful you will be in keeping your attitude steady and positive.

To use this strategy:

This strategy works well with the double-column technique in your Coping Notebook. On the left side, write down thoughts you have that reflect a negative attitude about your illness. Then on the right side, write down what someone else would say, someone who has a more positive mental attitude about living with their condition. (If you're not sure what they'd say, find people with positive mental attitudes and ask them!) Make sure the comments you write are realistic, or your mind won't accept them. Refer often to the answers you've written.

[ ] #122

Develop a Resilience Toolkit

When you're in the middle of a tough moment, it can be hard to remember what actually helps. A resilience toolkit gives you ready-to-use support.

Your toolkit can be simple—a folder, a box, or a note/app on your phone that holds things that reliably help you feel steadier. These can be songs, photos, quotes, relaxation exercises (or links), or names of people you trust when you need to reach out.

To use this strategy:

Think of your toolkit as a personalized collection of strategies and ideas that can help you when you need them. To put it together, try the following:

- Make a list of coping strategies that you know help you calm down or regain balance.
- Store tangible items (journal, printed quotes, written affirmations, links to relaxation exercises) together in one place you can reach quickly.
- Practice using these tools on easier days, so they'll feel familiar when stress levels increase.
- Review and update your toolkit periodically, adding or removing items as you need

[ ] #123

Use Positive Affirmations

A great way to help you improve your attitude is to use positive affirmations. These are short, encouraging statements you say aloud or silently to yourself. They are designed to strengthen you, help you think more positively, believe in yourself, and counter automatic negative thoughts.

By repeating these affirmations, they can become an ongoing part of your thinking. Even if you don't believe them at first, if they are realistic and you'd like to believe them, repetition can make them part of how you think.

Affirmations aren't about denying difficult feelings. Acknowledge what's hard and then pair it with a helpful statement (e.g., "This is hard, and I can take the next small step.").

Effective affirmations are short, believable, present-tense, and aligned with your values. Avoid all-or-nothing or unrealistic claims; soften with phrases like "I can...," "I'm learning to...," or "I choose to...," so your mind accepts them. Examples you can use or modify include: "I can take one small step today." "I deserve care and support." "I can ask for help when I need it." "Even on hard days, I can breathe and steady myself." "I can handle this appointment."

Try to use them at regularly scheduled times, such as morning or bedtime, before/after appointments, during flare-ups, and any time you notice self-criticism. In your Coping Notebook, keep a "Top 5" list and note which affirmations help most; review and revise monthly.

To use this strategy:

Here's a simple way to start and sustain the habit:

- In your Coping Notebook, list 3–5 realistic statements you truly want to believe.
- Say each line out loud; if one feels false, soften it (e.g., "I'm learning to...").

- Put them where you'll see them (sticky notes, lock screen) or record them in your voice.
- Link each repetition to a daily cue (morning meds, before appointments, during flare-ups) and pair it with one calming breath or a small behavior (taking medication, sipping water).

For example: "I'm working on small steps that help me manage my condition." "This is a difficult time, and I'm continuing the strategies that help me feel better."

Then, commit to reading them or, preferably, saying them, out loud, to yourself, a minimum of three times a day. Saying them aloud helps— you're reading, speaking, and hearing them. (Use a whisper or silent repeat when you're in public!)

Remember: repetition is what makes this strategy work. Keep at it, and affirmations will become more and more a part of your natural way of thinking.

[ ] #124

Change Pessimism to Optimism

Has some pessimism crept into your thinking following your diagnosis? That's common. Your thinking might become unusually negative, or you may worry about your future. This can certainly interfere with your efforts to accept and adapt to your diagnosis.

It makes sense to try to change pessimistic thoughts to more realistic, optimistic thoughts. The key word is realistic. For example, it might sound optimistic to say, "My chronic illness is going to go away," but is that truly realistic, or wishful thinking?

To use this strategy:

Use your Coping Notebook with the double-column technique to work on changing your thinking:

- Left column: Write the exact pessimistic thought as you notice it.
- Right column: Rewrite it in a realistic, optimistic way (what you might say to a friend in your situation).
- Read and repeat: Say the new version out loud and refer back to it if the old thought returns.

So, for example, instead of saying, "The doctor will never figure out how to control my symptoms" (a pessimistic thought), you might say, "Why should I convince myself of that? The doctor is trying very hard. I'm going to keep trying too." (More realistic and helpful.)

WHAT'S NEXT?

You may feel that you'll never be the same. But you are still the person you were before the diagnosis. Even if there is now a new reality in your life that may lead to some changes in what you do and how you feel, you are still you. Be positive ... about your life... and about yourself.

The next chapter offers strategies to help you become a better participant in your self-care, both physically and emotionally.

CHAPTER 8

I Need to Support My Body Wisely

In the last chapter, you read about strategies to help strengthen your inner self. Now, let's turn to your body. Regardless of how your illness affects you, you still need to care for your body. Every small step you take to support your physical well-being can help you living well after diagnosis.

This chapter offers practical strategies to improve your nutrition, build strength and stamina safely, reduce stress, sleep better, and conserve energy—and to make healthy choices about tobacco, alcohol, and other habits. Always check with your medical team before making significant changes, since some recommendations may need to be tailored to your specific condition.

The theme for this chapter is simple: make good choices, more often. You don't need to be perfect—no one is. If you slip, notice it, learn from it, forgive yourself, and move on. Use your Coping Notebook to track what works. Pick one small change and start there.

[ ] #125

Improve Your Nutrition

Good nutrition helps your energy, strength, recovery, and symptom control. When you eat well, your body can be stronger, more energized, and better able to handle your condition. Some symptoms may improve with dietary changes—check with your medical team before you adjust your plan.

Some conditions need quick changes; others do better with small, steady steps. A balanced plan that you can stick with is best.

Try to follow the most widely accepted nutritional guidelines, unless otherwise directed by your medical team. For example: eat a variety of foods; choose vegetables, fruits, whole grains, and lean protein; limit sugar, salty foods, and alcohol; drink water; smaller, more frequent meals may help; ask your doctor or a registered dietitian before taking supplements.

Again, these are suggestions showing some of the many things you can do. You should, however, clear everything with your medical team. Some of the most widely accepted suggestions as set forth above may be contraindicated, or even dangerous, if you've been diagnosed with certain conditions. Until you do, take any nutritional advice with a grain of (low-sodium) salt!

To use this strategy:

Determine the foods and eating behaviors that are inappropriate for you, or not in your best interest. Use your double-column technique in your Coping Notebook to make a list of them on the left side of the page. Add to the list as you become aware of any new ones. On the right side, decide and write down the changes you want (or need) to make (either to implement more appropriate behaviors, or to reduce or eliminate the inappropriate ones).

In addition, if you're experiencing any symptoms that can be helped by nutritional modifications, include that as well. If you do make helpful changes to your diet, write down how you feel after making these adjustments. This type of positive reinforcement can motivate you to continue your efforts.

Don't feel that all alterations must be made at once. Set up a timetable for making changes and record your progress. Be sure any changes you make include good nutritional common sense (and don't hesitate to reach out to healthcare professionals if you have any questions or concerns).

[ ] #126
Stop Smoking

Smoking is hazardous to your health. So, eliminating it is an important part of any self-improvement program. If you're smoking, stop! (Big shock!) If you don't smoke, you can move on to the next strategy!

At the time of this writing, I'm not aware of any chronic illnesses that are enhanced by smoking, so why do it? Yes, it may be difficult to stop. (Remember the words of Mark Twain: "Giving up smoking is the easiest thing in the world. I know, because I've done it thousands of times.") But if your goal is to enhance your health following your diagnosis, make it your business to do this ... soon!

If you want to do this by yourself, go for it. But you don't have to stop smoking on your own. If you feel that you need some support, there are many good healthcare experts who can help you, as well as books, articles, professional programs, and assistive devices that you can use to stop.

If you vape, talk with your doctor or nurse about what's safest for you. Some people use vaping for a short time for prescribed reasons. Others are advised to stop. Make a plan that fits your health needs.

Do some research, speak to your doctor, and then set a target date by which you plan to be a non-smoker.

To use this strategy:

Set up a page in your Coping Notebook for your stop-smoking efforts. Include notes about the following on your page:

- Write down your reasons for smoking and then counteract them. Also, include your reasons for wanting to quit.
- Set a realistic quit date and write it in your Coping Notebook.
- Determine your plan for how you're going to stop smoking. Write it out, step by step, with a tentative timetable.
- Then make a commitment. Commit to your goal to stop smoking by signing a contract (with yourself, or a significant other).
- Clear your space. Remove cigarettes/vapes, lighters, ashtrays, and other cues.
- Use the double-column technique- on the left side, write your triggers (coffee, stress, driving); on the right side, write what you'll do instead (wait 10 minutes, breathe, sip water, short walk, text a friend).
- Write down substitutes you can grab fast (gum, mints, water, cut fruit/veggies) and write simple calming tools (slow breaths, stretch, brief walk) that you'd use.
- Plan (and write) other (healthy) substitute activities.
- Give yourself rewards for stopping.

Check off each step as you accomplish it. Nothing motivates as much as success.

[ ] #127

Control Your Alcohol Intake

Although drinking is not the no-no that smoking is, obviously moderation is essential. In addition, the possible dangerous interactions between alcohol and some of the medications that may be part of your treatment will help to determine how important it is to control your drinking.

Your doctor is the best person to tell you how much, if any, you can safely drink. After all, your goal is to help your body, so why do anything that could interfere with that?

(Obviously, if you have problems with alcohol or other substances, that goes beyond the focus of this strategy. This is certainly something that needs to be addressed as part of your self-improvement efforts, and you should consult with your treatment team to get moving with this.)

To use this strategy:

In your Coping Notebook, write out a plan to be in control of your alcohol consumption. You may want to determine how often or how much you drink, what you'll drink, and when. The more specific your goals and the steps you'll follow to achieve them, the more likely it is that you'll succeed.

You may find it helpful, if not essential, to run your goals by your doctor to make sure you're both on the same page. Then implement your plan and get high on knowing that this is another solid way that you're helping yourself!

[ ] #128

Get Enough Exercise

Exercise is one of the most effective ways to improve your health. It's a natural outlet for your body, a great way to strengthen your physical self, and a healthy way to release stressful energy.

Research has actually shown that exercise can help people deal with many of the symptoms of chronic illnesses, including pain! That's why it makes sense to talk with your doctor about what you can do safely, and then set up a plan to make exercise part of your coping program.

Exercise will help your body both physically and psychologically. Some of the benefits include:

- Helping to energize your body
- Helping you to defuse stress or other negative emotions
- Strengthening your self-confidence and improving your body image
- Helping you to sleep better
- Helping your overall physical and mental health

There are always types of exercise you can do, regardless of how your symptoms may be limiting you. You do need to avoid anything that could be unsafe for your condition. Even if you can only exercise part of your body because of limitations, it's better than not doing anything.

To use this strategy:

Start by getting advice from your doctor as to what kinds of exercise, and how much of it, you can or cannot do. This consultation is critical, especially in the early stages of living with your condition. You don't want to hurt yourself, but because exercise is so valuable, you also don't want to leave it out of your life.

Write out a plan for your exercise routine. Include what you're going to do, how long, and how often. Note any questions that you have about your program so you can discuss them with your doctor.

Begin gradually. Doing too much too soon can backfire, especially if you're out of shape. You'll either end up losing interest or even injure yourself. (Either way, you'll hurt!) Start slowly but steadily, and increase as your body allows.

Pace yourself. You've heard the phrase, "No pain, no gain." That may not apply to you. Consider low-impact activities-- examples include walking and swimming—are often good choices. If you can do more, you might try cycling. These kinds of activities can actually strengthen muscles, reduce pain, and decrease stiffness. (More about pacing in Strategy #135.)

The most important final note about exercising? Stick with it. Starting and stopping doesn't bring the same benefits as being consistent. Jot down how you feel after you exercise. This can be a motivation to continue doing it.

[ ] #129

Strengthen Yourself with Gentle Motion

If the word "exercise" feels exhausting, think instead about "gentle movement." Gentle movement strengthens your body without overexertion and builds a healthier mind-body connection. Simple activities like yoga, tai chi, stretching, or short walks can improve flexibility, circulation, balance, and mood. Best of all, they can be adjusted to your energy level on any given day.

To use this strategy:

Start by asking your healthcare team what types of gentle movement are safe for you right now. Once you know what's appropriate, begin with short sessions—five to ten minutes is plenty to get started. You can use beginner videos online, books, or community classes to guide you, especially if you're new to practices like yoga or tai chi.

Increase your activity slowly and give yourself credit for every bit of progress. Even small efforts count. If all you can manage one day is a short stretch or a slow walk around the room, that's still movement. The important thing is to listen to your body, go at your own pace, and notice the benefits. Over time, you may find these gentle practices become a steady, enjoyable part of your routine.

[ ] #130

Get Enough Rest

One of the most important things you can do to help yourself is to get enough rest (and sleep). This is true no matter what your condition may be. The good news is that it's relatively easy to make this a regular part of your daily routine.

Each person has a finite amount of energy each day. Research suggests that people with chronic illnesses often have less. Therefore, more rest may be necessary to rejuvenate your energy. Rest also supports your immune system and allows your body to balance activity with recovery.

Why is this so important? You're trying to do everything you can to help yourself deal with your condition, right? This chapter is focused on strategies for improving your physical well-being. Well, getting enough rest needs to be added to that list.

It's important to learn how much rest you need. Learn how to hear what your body is saying. Don't push too much. Build in periodic rest times throughout the day, whenever you know your body needs it.

It will take time to truly know the balance of activity, rest, and sleep that works for you. You'll only learn this by experience. Stay on top of this. It's a simple but essential way of supporting yourself as you deal with your diagnosis and its effects.

To use this strategy:

In your Coping Notebook, create a page just for rest and sleep. Keep track of what you learn about how much rest you need. This may change from day to day, but patterns will emerge over time.

Jot down when you notice the need to rest, how long you rest, and which activities make you more tired. Note how much sleep seems best for you at night. Add any ideas that help you weave rest into your routine, so it becomes a natural part of your self-care.

[ ] #131

Improve Your Sleeping Habits

Sleep difficulties can be part of your illness—and they can also make your symptoms harder to manage. There are many ways to improve your sleep routine. Here are just a few examples. In the evening, before going to bed, you might try:

- Not eating close to bedtime (unless medically necessary)
- Avoiding stimulants like caffeine or certain medicines, if possible
- Keeping activity light—no vigorous exercise right before bed
- Lowering the lights in your room
- Turning off electronic devices at least 30 minutes before sleep

To use this strategy:

In your Coping Notebook, write down the specific sleep problems you notice—for example, tossing and turning when you first get into bed. Beside each one, note the tip or strategy you'll try, such as listening to a relaxation recording. If you suspect your medications may play a role, write down questions to ask your doctor or pharmacist.

After trying each strategy, record the results—for instance, "slept more soundly than usual." Add your own suggestions as you learn what works best. Over time, you'll build a personal guide to better sleep.

[ ] #132
Reduce Stress

This strategy seems like a no-brainer, right? But it's worth saying clearly: every health problem can be helped by reducing stress.

Stress is something that affects everyone. The degree of stress is what determines whether it's a normal part of life, or potentially harmful.

Stress comes from many sources, and these vary from person to person. Given how important it is to control stress—no matter what you've been diagnosed with—it makes sense to do everything you can to manage it. And the good news is that this is something you can start working on right away.

To use this strategy:

In your Coping Notebook, start a "stress page." Begin by asking yourself: "What exactly is causing me stress?" Try to pinpoint the main sources.

For example, your stress may be related to your diagnosis, your symptoms, medication side effects, doctor visits, how your illness limits your activities, or how it affects others around you. Your illness-related list could go on and on. Write down anything that comes to mind. Then add stressors not directly related to your illness—things that may have already been affecting you before your diagnosis.

Once you have started pinpointing your stressors, start writing down goals for how you'll reduce them. Create a step-by-step plan for what you'll try. Use the pinpointing and goal-setting strategies in Chapter 4 (Strategies #70 and #71) to formulate a clear, workable plan.

Then, get started. Everything you do to reduce your stress can help your body and mind. Keep track of your progress in your notebook and adjust your plan along the way. Add new ideas as you discover them.

If you have difficulty accomplishing your stress reduction goals, consider working with a professional who can help you with stress management. This can be a big help!

[ ] #133
Explore Stress-Reducing Hobbies

Hobbies bring joy and calm, and they remind you that you are more than your illness. When illness tries to take center stage, hobbies—painting, music, gardening, crafts, puzzles, or countless others—shift your focus to something creative and satisfying. They provide balance, pleasure, and even a sense of connection with others.

To use this strategy:

Start by choosing an activity you already enjoy, or one you've always wanted to try. It doesn't have to be big or complicated—what matters most is that it feels good to you. Once you've picked something, set aside a short, regular block of time for it. Consistency matters more than duration, so even ten minutes a day can be a good way to start. Adjust the activity to match your energy level. For example, on low-energy days, you might simply sketch, knit a few rows, or tend to one plant. On better days, you may want to do more.

If you'd like to add a social benefit, share your hobby with others. Join a group class, trade recipes with a friend, or post a picture of your project. In your Coping Notebook, jot down which hobbies you try and how they make you feel. Over time, you'll build a personal list of activities that lower your stress and lift your spirits.

[ ] #134

Know Your Limitations

It's very important to focus on what you can do, rather than dwelling on what you can't—or shouldn't—do.

Your activities may be limited by any of your symptoms or physical restrictions, such as pain and fatigue. Knowing your limitations will also help you pace yourself (see the next strategy). It will help you to be as productive as possible during your day.

Yes, you may need to make some changes, as compared to what you could or could not do prior to your diagnosis. But the goal is not to feel unhappy about these changes. Instead, it's to feel good about the things you *are* able to do. Focus on that and, hopefully, you'll be able to do more.

[ ] #135

Be Active, but Pace Yourself

It's always good to be as active as you can be. But you have to create a good balance between being active (expending energy) and resting (replenishing your energy). That balance is what pacing is all about.

It can sometimes be helpful to carve out a particular time of day for rest. You will most likely learn this by experience. For example, if you know that your motor is winding down by mid-afternoon, that may be the best time to schedule a rest break.

Make pacing yourself a conscious part of your routine. Don't hesitate to share your pacing plan with family and friends. They will respect your needs and will hopefully be supportive. They may even decide to plan their own rest times as well!

To use this strategy:

In your Coping Notebook, keep a page for pacing. Jot down the times of day you most often feel tired, and how long a rest break seems to help. This may take time to figure out, and can always change.

As you experiment, jot down what works best: alternating activity and rest, slowing down your pace, breaking a large task into smaller steps, or other strategies. When something unexpected disrupts your routine, don't blame yourself. Just revise your schedule and try again.

[ ] #136

Take Time for Yourself

No matter how much you have to do, no matter how much you're trying to learn, and no matter how you feel, you always want (and need!) to take time for yourself. This is not a luxurious self-indulgence. Think of it as a healthy necessity. Taking personal time restores balance, brings enjoyment, and keeps your life from being consumed by illness.

Your goal is to create a healthy balance between the things that you have to do and the things that you want to do. You know the saying "all work and no play…"? Well, that applies here, too. No matter how busy your schedule is, and no matter how you feel physically, make sure you establish some time each day (even if it's a short time) for something you enjoy that relaxes you.

Some examples? You might read, listen to music, watch your favorite show, sit outside in fresh air, take a walk, do needlework, take a bubble bath, color, call a friend, or do a puzzle. The activity doesn't matter as much as the fact that it feels good and gives you a break.

To use this strategy:

In your Coping Notebook, make a list of relaxing activities you enjoy. These don't need to be complicated. Anything that brings a smile or a sense of calm belongs on the list. Once you've got a few ideas written down, choose one or two each day and plan when you'll do them.

You might notice patterns: some activities help when you're tired, others when you're stressed or restless. Write those observations in your notebook so you'll know what to reach for in different situations. Over time, you'll build a personal menu of go-to activities that help keep your days in balance.

[ ] #137

Conserve Energy

Because you've been diagnosed with a condition that is affecting your body, it makes sense to conserve as much energy as possible—saving it for things that matter most. This doesn't mean you should be lazy; it means you're looking for ways to make life easier for yourself. Conserving energy reduces fatigue and helps you accomplish more with less stress.

To use this strategy:

Think about your day as a limited supply of energy that you need to spend wisely. In your Coping Notebook, write down tasks that seem to drain you more than they should. Next to each one, write down ideas for how you might handle them differently to conserve your energy.

For example, you might choose clothing that's easier to put on and take off. You could use gadgets or tools that make routine tasks quicker. You may decide to cut out activities that aren't important, reduce the energy you expend in routine activities, or spread out heavier tasks over several days instead of doing them all at once. And, of course, remember to include rest periods in your daily routine.

Track how you feel after making these changes. Notice which adjustments help most, and keep adding new ones as you discover them. Over time, conserving energy in small ways can leave you with more strength for the things that really matter to you.

[ ] #138
Make Changes in Your Living Environment

People may not be aware of the degree to which their physical surroundings can play an important role in how well they live following their diagnosis. Everything you can do to make things easier and more comfortable at home can help you to conserve energy, enabling you to spend it on more important things. Creating an environment that supports you reduces fatigue and stress, and helps you get more done with less effort.

Examples of changes you can make in your living environment include installing new, easier-to-use doorknobs or cabinet handles, reorganizing your home to make things more easily accessible, using a dehumidifier to make air quality more comfortable, and so much more. Even small changes can make your daily life less draining.

You can learn more about this by reading about how your living environment may affect your condition, or by seeking advice from your doctor or other people who understand your needs.

To use this strategy:

Take a fresh look at your surroundings. Walk through your home with your Coping Notebook (or a clipboard and paper) and jot down ideas for how to make things more comfortable and easier for you. Pay special attention to tasks that once felt automatic but now cause strain or discomfort.

Next, think of simple adjustments that could make those tasks easier—moving heavy pans to a lower shelf, adding brighter lighting in a hallway, or keeping often-used items close at hand. You don't have to make all the changes at once. Start with one or two that could give you quick relief.

Over time, keep adding to your list and updating it. Each small change you make helps your home become more "you-friendly," conserving your energy and making daily life smoother.

WHAT'S NEXT?

There are many other things you can do to improve your physical well-being, from a relaxing massage to a refreshing vacation. The most important point is this: there are always steps you can take, large or small, to help your body cope better with illness.

In the next chapter, we'll shift from focusing on your body to focusing on your connections—how to strengthen relationships and build a support network that will help you living well despite your diagnosis.

CHAPTER 9

I Need to Strengthen My Circle of Support

In the time following your diagnosis, it is important not to isolate yourself. Instead, make sure to reach out for support. Getting support from family and friends is invaluable. No one should have to face illness alone.

Research indicates that people who try to manage a chronic illness by themselves have a harder time adjusting and moving forward.

A strong support system can help you handle challenges, lift your spirits, and provide both practical and emotional assistance. Your support system may include family, friends, coworkers, health professionals, and community members. The goal is to surround yourself with people who understand, encourage, and help you living well after diagnosis.

This chapter offers strategies to build, strengthen, and maintain your support system so you can feel less isolated and more empowered on your journey.

A- Who Should Be on Your Support Team?

We've discussed strategies for setting up and working with your medical team. Now let's talk more about your personal support team.

The more people you interact with, the less alone you will feel. Having a variety of people in your network also makes it more likely that when you need someone to listen, to talk with, or to help you, there will be somebody available. In addition, the more people you have in your support network, the more you'll be able to "spread out" the potentially difficult, time-consuming, or even draining responsibilities of being supportive to your needs.

It's also easier for different people to help in different ways than for any one person to feel as though you're depending on them for everything. Family, friends, neighbors, coworkers, members of your faith community, and peers who share similar health experiences can all be part of your team.

[ ] #139

Select Individuals for Your Support Team

Everyone has different people in their lives, and they may play different roles. Here we're focusing on the *non-professionals* in your life. For example, before you were diagnosed, you'd know who you might want to go to a movie with, who you would call to go out to eat with, and who to talk to if you had a problem with your kids.

Think about each of the people in your life that you'd like to be on your support team. You'll likely have a good idea which of them will be more receptive to supporting you, and in what ways. Think of the role that each one can play, and how you're going to approach them about being on your team.

Your support team should include those people whom you can most easily lean on when necessary. They should build you up, rather than add to your stress. Try to surround yourself with positive, inspirational, upbeat, supportive individuals. You want to draw as much strength as you can from them. Your go-to people should be the ones you trust, can talk to, and believe will be there for you.

The more people you have around you who fit these qualities, the more support you likely can count on. It also spreads the effort so no one person feels overwhelmed.

To use this strategy:

In your Coping Notebook, start a page called "My Support Team." Begin by writing a simple list of people you might reach out to, for any reason. This list can change over time. Next to each name, note their strengths (good listener, rides, tech help, meal help, childcare), how they prefer to be contacted (text, call, email), and when they're usually available. This gives you a quick picture of who might help with what.

Think about the role each person could play and when you would reach out. For example, you might ask a neighbor for a short grocery run, a friend for a check-in call after appointments, or a relative for rides. Be clear and realistic in what you ask, and use specific requests ("Could you drive me on Tuesday at 2 PM?") so it's easy to say yes.

Plan backups so you don't overload anyone. For each need, jot down two or three options you could contact. If someone can't help, you'll have another choice ready. For each need, list two or three options you could contact. If someone can't help, you'll have another choice ready. Update your page as you learn who is most comfortable with which tasks, and remember to thank people and rotate requests so your team stays strong.

[ ] #140
Limit Exposure to Negativity

Because you're dealing with the stress of your diagnosis, be selective about who you spend time with. Some, as you know, will be supportive. Others, however, may not be. They may, either purposely or not, make life more difficult for you.

Letting go of or keeping more distance from "toxic" or consistently negative people who provide you with more hassle than support is a valuable coping strategy. Be aware of those people who cause you more stress. Then reduce, limit, or, if needed, eliminate contact with them.

This need not be a permanent change. Relationships and feelings change. But this is an important way to make sure you're taking care of yourself. You can always reassess later.

Obviously, there are times when some "downers" are in the "unavoidable" category. When this happens, focus instead on how you'll better deal with them to minimize any negative impact they may have. Short visits, neutral topics, and clear "end times" can help.

To use this strategy:

In your Coping Notebook, start a page called "Contact Comfort Plan" for this strategy. Write the initials or a brief description (for privacy) of anyone whose presence feels more draining than supportive. Jot down why you feel this way and what boundary might help (shorter visits, fewer calls, different topics, or taking a break from contact).

Plan gentle, clear wording you can use with them when needed—for example: "I'm keeping my stress low right now, so I need to keep this short," or "I'm not talking about medical details today. Let's talk about something lighter." If contact is unavoidable, set a start and end time, choose a neutral setting, and have an exit plan (another appointment, a planned rest). Revisit your page monthly and adjust as relationships shift.

[ ] #141

Understand the Discomfort That Others May Feel

There are times when you may not get the support you want from some family members or friends, as much as you may want it. Some just may not be able to deal with what you're going through. They may be scared when they are told a loved one has an illness. They may not know how to handle their own feelings, let alone be there for you.

When this happens, there are often reasons for their discomfort. Try not to take it personally. (Yes, this is easier said than done.) It most likely has less to do with you, and more to do with them.

Why does this happen? Significant others may identify with your current situation. In other words, what you're going through is upsetting to them. They may have a hard time thinking about how *they* would deal with such a diagnosis, and therefore don't want to think about it. So, they may not be as supportive of you because that would make it hard to push it out of their minds.

Others may not have the patience to be there for you in ways they think you'll need it. Or they may have difficulty seeing you as different from the way you were before your diagnosis. Still others may not even believe that you're sick, especially if you look healthy.

Remember, this doesn't mean that they don't love you or care about you. It may just mean that their own fears or unhelpful ways of thinking have blocked them from being supportive in the ways you'd like (and possibly even in the ways they'd like).

Whatever the reason(s), it's not worth pushing someone to be supportive. Being understanding (as much as you can be) may give them the space to deal with their own discomforts and ultimately feel more at ease with the situation. They may see that you're still basically the same person you were, and they may realize that your being diagnosed doesn't mean that this will happen to them. If they come around, that will be a plus for you. (This is especially true if you don't close the door and eliminate them from your life because they're initially unable to be supportive.)

For those who are just not able to deal with your condition, accept it, and put your energy into others who *will* be supportive in the ways you want … and deserve. You deserve a team that helps you feel safer and stronger.

To use this strategy:

In your Coping Notebook, write the names or initials of people whose support feels uncertain. Next to each, note a possible reason for their discomfort (fear, not knowing what to say, denial, seeing you as you were before). This reminder can help you take it less personally.

Plan a simple next step for each person: a short update, a specific request ("Could you text me on treatment days?"), or a gentle boundary ("I'm avoiding scary stories about illness—can we talk about something else?"). If someone continues to struggle, lower your expectations, keep conversations brief and neutral, and leave the door open: "If you want to talk later, I'm here."

Finally, shift your energy toward the people who can show up now. Add those names to your Support Team page and keep building the network that helps you most.

[ ] #142
Be Prepared for the Reactions of Others

It is said that the best way to determine the people who truly care about you is to go through a crisis. Your medical condition can feel like that kind of crisis.

You'll quickly determine the people who are supportive and willing to help, and the people who seem to move away from you. Unfortunately, this is inevitable. Not everyone will be fully understanding or support-ive, and it's up to you how much you let this affect you.

Obviously, none of the significant people in your life, family or friends, are going to be happy that you've been diagnosed with a chronic illness. But you may fear that people, even ones close to you, may distance themselves from you because of your diagnosis. And in some cases, this may happen.

Hopefully, you'll be pleasantly surprised at how they can and will rally around you. Sharing simple, clear information about what you're going through may make this easier.

Try not to have expectations of how some people will react. You don't want to be devastated if they're not there for you.

Comfort yourself by remembering, realistically, that not all people can or will react exactly the way you'd hope they would. Then you can focus your energy on enjoying the support and attention from those who continue to be supportive.

To use this strategy:

Take a little time to plan how you'll explain your diagnosis and what kind of support helps. In your Coping Notebook, jot down a few notes about what you want to say and how much detail you want to share with different people. You may explain the same facts in different ways for different people—short and simple for some, a bit more detail for others. Prepare a one- or two-sentence update you can use when you need help, such as: "I'm dealing with [condition]. What I really need right now is [specific help], and I'll share more when I have the energy."

Think about some of the initial ways that you might want support— for example, a ride, a check-in text, help with a task, or just company. Practice a gentle boundary for conversations that feel uncomfortable, such as: "I don't want to talk about scary stories today—could we switch topics?" After you talk with people, write down how each person reacts and any next steps. This helps you take things less personally, keep doors open where it makes sense, and spend more time with the people who show up.

[ ] #143

Be Aware of the Most Important Member of Your Support Team

Guess who that is? You're right ... it's you!

You are the coordinator of your team. You're the center of the support wheel. The best way for you to benefit from the support of others is to keep noticing the strength you still have and use it to organize the help you need.

You've been diagnosed with a chronic illness. Yes, there are ways that your life will change, but the basic you is still in there. You're not broken. Don't let yourself feel that you are.

An important goal following your diagnosis is to be able to support yourself. Obviously, the more you can do for yourself, the better. But there is no shame in benefiting from the help of others. Your strength plus their support is the combination you're aiming for.

B- Plan and Expand Your Support

Now that we have discussed how to put together your support team, let's discuss ways of dealing with and interacting with them. This section will offer strategies, including how to work with them day to day, how to ask for specific help, set ground rules, coordinate tasks, and keep support going over time.

[ ] #144

Be Able to Explain Your Illness to Others

Many people—some caring, some curious, some unsure, and some skeptical—will ask you about your physical condition. You want to know how to respond, and how to briefly explain it to them.

Whether it's family, friends, acquaintances, colleagues, employers, or others, you want to be able to explain what you've learned about your disease following your diagnosis. It helps to organize a few key facts as you learn them. Being prepared to share a very brief, basic summary of what you know, and how it's affecting you, can help you when you want or need to explain it to someone. How much you share depends on the person and the moment.

To use this strategy:

In your Coping Notebook, write down short answers to the common questions you may hear, including:

- What exactly is ________________ (your condition)?
- How were you diagnosed?
- How does it affect you (your symptoms)?
- What is the treatment? Who are you working with?
- What additional information is important for others to know about your condition (e.g., is it contagious?)

You'll feel better knowing that you're ready to provide information about your condition, how it affects you, and what is being done about it. Keep it simple and in your own words.

Then draft a one- or two-sentence version for days you're low on energy (e.g., "I'm managing [condition]. Right now, it mainly affects [symptom]. I'm working with [clinician/team]."). Share only what you're comfortable sharing. Jot down new questions people ask so you can add them later and fill in any gaps in what you know.

[ ] #145

Set Ground Rules

There are times when significant others may not be as supportive as you'd like, or may not know how to meet your needs. They may not understand your condition, how you're affected by it, or what your needs are. Often, they'll move further away from you, rather than risk upsetting you by doing the wrong thing.

The best way to try to make this as easy as possible for everyone (including yourself!) is to set ground rules. Setting ground rules, letting others know exactly what you need or prefer from them, can improve relationships by eliminating questions or confusion. Clear, kind guidelines—what helps and what doesn't—reduce confusion and make support easier.

For example, if there are times you don't want to talk about your condition, say so. Tell them that there may be times when you don't want to talk about it, and you would appreciate their sensitivity and consideration when you feel that way. At the same time, let them know that when you feel better, you'll be happy to talk with them.

Setting ground rules is not about controlling everything. Rather, it's your way of being aware of how you feel physically, how you feel emotionally—when you feel like talking and when you don't, when need help and when you don't—and how to communicate this to others.

This is also not about you being cold or insensitive. If anything, this is an effort to make things more comfortable for everyone. In fact, in many cases, significant others want to know what you'd prefer. They may be looking to you for those ground rules, so that they will know how to be there for you.

To use this strategy:

Think ahead about what would make interactions easier. You may have a few general rules for everyone (e.g., "Please text before calling," "No scary stories about illness") and some specific ones that are for certain people (e.g., "Short visits work best," "Please help with rides, not medical advice"). In your Coping Notebook, note the person or group, the situation that prompted the need for a ground rule, and what you'd like to try.

Plan how you'll say these ground rules—when, where, and how. You'll want to keep them mainly short and kind. For example: "I'm keeping medical talk brief right now. If you want to help, a check-in text after appointments is great." or "I'm not discussing test details today—could we talk about something lighter?"

Finally, anticipate any reactions, comments, or suggestions that might be uncomfortable for you. This will help you to better prepare for them, and, hopefully, soothe any ruffled feathers.

[ ] #146

Be Able to Ask for Help

Following your diagnosis, you'll learn from experience what you're able to do and what you are less able to do. This may change as you feel better (or worse), depending on changes in your symptoms or condition.

Should you ask for help from others? Why not? Would you be upset if someone asked you for help? You probably would not hesitate. So why not? Most people are glad to help when they know what you need.

This may be especially difficult if asking for help is not something you're accustomed to. Some people say it's the first time in their life that they've ever had to ask for help. This is often one of the hardest things to do after a diagnosis. Remember, there is nothing wrong with this. It's a way to help you improve your situation.

If you ask for help, either you'll get it or you won't. If you don't ask, you won't know. This is information that's important to know for the future. Obviously, your goal is not to take advantage (or be seen as taking advantage). In fact, you may want to mention your concerns about taking advantage, and even ask your friends or loved ones to let you know if they think you're ever overstepping.

There may be times when you're pleasantly surprised by others (often, people you did not expect) asking you if you need help. (That's SO much easier than you having to ask them, right?) Take advantage of that opportunity ... but don't take advantage of them. Look at this as a win-win. You'll get the help you need, and they'll feel good about being able to help. Start slowly with what you ask of them. Be realistic, be fair, and be appreciative.

To use this strategy:

First, in your Coping Notebook, identify the specific things you can't currently do, or would like help doing. Then, jot down ideas about one or two people who might be a good fit.

Then, plan your approach: when you'll ask and what you'll say. Ask calmly, be appreciative, and accept "no" without taking it personally. If asking feels uncomfortable, remind yourself you'd want them to feel safe asking you, too.

[ ] #147

Choose an "Information Manager"

There is so much information out there that you'll quickly feel overwhelmed trying to learn everything you can about your condition.

Then add the well-intentioned comments and suggestions that arrive from nearly everyone who hears about your diagnosis.

Be aware of when you get to the point of feeling stressed or worn out trying to digest all of this information. If you do, ask a family member or friend if they would be willing to be your "information manager". With your permission, you can forward articles, links, and advice to this person—or ask others to share tips directly with them. Your helper filters it, keeps what's relevant, and brings you a short, useful summary so you can decide what to act on (or ignore).

To use this strategy:

Write a brief "information manager" note in your Coping Notebook: who you'll ask, why you chose them, and what you're asking them to do. When you invite them, explain the role in simple terms ("I get overwhelmed by all the information. Could I send articles to you, and you send me a short summary of what matters?").

Agree on how to share items (email, text, shared folder, snail mail), how often to check in (for example, weekly), and what to prioritize (doctor-approved sources, treatment updates, side-effect tips). Set boundaries about what you do and don't want to read, and ask them to flag urgent items only. If they let you know it's become too much, add a backup helper or narrow the scope so it stays manageable.

[ ] #148

Keep Track of the Nice Things That People Do for You

It can be very helpful to keep track of the nice things that people do for you. This will help you remember the kinds of things that you can reach out to them for, and the ways that they can help you.

It will also help you make sure that you acknowledge the things that they do. Not only will their acts of kindness be helpful to you, but the emotional support you derive from their assistance will help your coping efforts. Seeing these notes in one place can also lift your mood on hard days.

To use this strategy:

In your Coping Notebook, keep track of any acts of kindness that you experience. Include the date, the person, what they did, and how you acknowledged it (text, note, call). Supportive gestures can be tangible (shopping, walking the dog, a helpful gift), or intangible (a caring phone call, a ride, sitting with you). Add a simple follow-up plan—when you might thank them again, return a favor, or ask for similar help in the future.

[ ] #149

Benefit from Healing Hugs (When Appropriate)

There are times when nonverbal communication is as good, if not better, than verbal communication. A perfect example of helpful nonverbal communication is a hug. It's a way of feeling close to a family member or friend, without saying anything. Hugs convey warmth, support, love, compassion, and a lot more.

Research suggests that hugs can be beneficial physiologically. They may lower blood pressure and can release oxytocin, a hormone linked with bonding and calmness. Also, hugs can be beneficial psychologically. They can reduce stress, and help you to feel cared about and less alone.

Don't always feel like you have to wait for somebody to volunteer a hug. There's nothing wrong with asking for one. Always make sure the other person is comfortable—consent matters.

Obviously, not everyone likes hugs. You'll want to be selective about when and who you ask for a hug. But try it. The warm, comforting feelings that result can only help!

[ ] #150

Learn from the Experiences of Others

Many people are comforted by hearing about the experiences of others who are living with the same or similar condition. This need not be limited to people you meet in a support group. You may hear, anywhere, first-person accounts of people living with your condition. For example, when a celebrity goes public because of a chronic illness, others with the same or similar condition often have a great deal of interest in hearing what this person has to say.

Many of these first-person accounts can be found by researching your condition online. Learning about others' successful experiences can be inspiring and reassuring. As always, keep your "reality filter" in place. Everyone's situation is different. Don't follow someone else's plan just because it worked for them. Talk with your medical team first.

To use this strategy:

In your Coping Notebook, keep a "Stories That Help" page. It may help you to keep a written record of any first-person anecdotes you hear about that seem helpful. By keeping these in your Coping Notebook, they will be a source of inspiration or support at those times when you may need them.

Jot down the source (book, video, post, talk), one or two takeaways that encouraged you, and any ideas to ask your clinician about. If something you read worries you, write it down too, and bring it up with your doctor. Over time, you'll build a short list of voices that will inspire you, and you'll stay grounded by checking ideas with your care team first.

C- Other Support Resources

There are many organizations and other resources that help people deal with chronic illness. This section offers simple ways to find additional support, including local groups, online communities, and professional services, so you can add the kinds of help that fit you best.

[ ] #151

Get Professional Support

Counseling can be invaluable for people who have been diagnosed with a chronic illness. It can be great to talk to a supportive, compassionate individual who is not emotionally involved in your life. You'll get encouragement and strategies for the issues that arise as a consequence of your diagnosis. This can be enormously helpful.

There are people who, before their diagnosis, never would've believed they would go for counseling. Even in this day and age, many people continue to look at this as a sign of weakness. This is far from the truth. Seeking help is a sign of strength. What you're really demonstrating is, "I want to feel better, and I'll take advantage of any resource that can help me."

Your therapist can be a very important part of your treatment and support team. Spend time researching who would be the best person for you. (See Strategy #110.) You can ask your physician, local health organization, or people in your support group for recommendations.

Regardless of the name(s) given to you, it's up to you to feel that "connection" and decide whether this person feels like a good fit.

Many professionals will talk to you on the phone or via video. This is especially helpful if you are physically unable to get to them, or if they have more experience with your condition than professionals who are geographically closer to you.

Be as selective in choosing a counselor as you would in choosing your physician. There can be a world of difference between the really good ones and the ones you would not want to spend time with.

You can also be selective in deciding when to speak to a counselor. There's no required frequency. You'll learn to judge when you might benefit from more regular appointments, as compared to when you can schedule "as needed" sessions. The twists and turns of your medical condition, as well as the ups and downs of your emotional state, will be the primary determining factors. (See Strategy #111 for more information about what to talk to your counselor about.)

To use this strategy:

Set up a page in the "treatment team" section of your Coping Notebook and list each professional you're considering (name, role, phone, email, address). Add where you heard about them, experience with your condition, approach (for example, CBT, supportive therapy), and cost and insurance coverage. Ask if they see people in person only, or also by phone or video. And jot down your first impression notes after the first call or session. Bring a short list of topics (see #111) to the first meeting. There's no one "right" schedule—use regular visits when you need steady support, and "as needed" check-ins when that fits better. If a fit isn't there, it's okay to try someone else (see #110).

[ ] #152

Get Involved with Organizations

In addition to building up your support team with people that you have known for a while, you can also include organizations that relate to your condition. Not only will you get valuable information from these organizations, but you'll feel very comforted knowing that the people in these individual groups are more likely to know exactly what you're going through and will be supportive in your coping efforts. Many also offer practical help—education, peer connections, navigation services, and sometimes financial assistance.

These days, almost every condition has a health organization devoted to it (some conditions have more than one). If your condition is rare, look for umbrella groups with similar symptoms or needs.

Ways to find these organizations include searching online, speaking to your doctors, or asking professionals in local hospitals, among others. You can also ask clinic social workers or patient navigators for reputable options.

To use this strategy:

In your Coping Notebook, make a page called "Organizations to Contact." List groups that might offer informational, emotional, social, practical, or financial support. Include names, websites, phone/email, a contact person if available, and what they provide (newsletters, helplines, webinars, grants, local chapters). Pick one or two to contact this week and jot down a simple script ("I'm newly diagnosed with [condition]; what resources do you recommend for getting started?"). Note what you learn and set a small next step (subscribe, attend a webinar, join a local chapter). This is an ongoing page—add and update as you go.

[ ] #153

Gain Support from a Support Group

Local support groups can be a great source of information and support. For many chronic illnesses, you can find condition-specific groups—locally or online. Joining one can be an important part of coping with your diagnosis. Two big benefits: you'll be around people who understand what you're going through (so you feel less alone), and you'll learn practical tips others have already found helpful.

Look for groups that are uplifting, respectful, and motivational, not ones that leave you feeling worse. The best groups are led by trained facilitators—professionals or qualified peers—who keep the conversation on track, steer away from unhelpful detours, and share useful tips and resources for living with your condition.

Once you find a group, give it time. It is often suggested that you attend at least three group meetings before deciding if this is the group for you. It also takes time to feel comfortable with new people.

Some people join online support groups. These can help if you're unable to find (or get to) an in-person location, or if you prefer less face-to-face contact. Make sure they're appropriate and well run—ideally affiliated with a health organization—and be mindful of privacy.

If your exact condition has no group, consider one for related conditions with similar challenges. It might not be as ideal as talking with people who have exactly what you have, but at least you'll be spending time with like-minded individuals, people who want to deal better with their conditions.

You can even talk to your doctor and ask if there are others being treated for your condition that might like to form or participate in a new support group.

To use this strategy:

On a page in your Coping Notebook, write down the names and contact information for any groups in your area (or online) that deal with your newly diagnosed condition. Write down the questions you want to ask of the facilitator, and, of course, include the answers you obtain to these questions.

On a page in your Coping Notebook, list local and online groups for your condition (or related ones). Add contact info, meeting times, whether there's a trained facilitator, and any notes about format (sharing, education, guest speakers), confidentiality, accessibility, and cost. Write a few questions to ask before attending (Who attends? How is the group run? What topics are typical?). After each meeting, jot down your impressions—how you felt afterward, what was helpful, what wasn't. Keep going to groups that leave you feeling supported and informed, and let go of those that don't fit.

[ ] #154

Benefit from Your Spirituality

Individuals who are religious may derive tremendous comfort, support, and connection from their spirituality as they cope with illness. If this is important to you, take advantage of the emotional support your spiritual beliefs can provide for you.

People feel differently about spirituality and coping: some are sure it helps, some don't find it helpful, and some aren't sure yet.

If you're in the first category, you likely already know what helps. Some people find that scheduling a regular period of time to engage in spiritual activities does add to their strength and ability to cope.

If you are an active member at a place of worship, your congregation and the activities there can be very helpful. Speaking to a member of the clergy can be encouraging as well. Many people say these connections lift their mood, help them feel less alone, and support a more hopeful outlook.

If you're in the second category, and this is not for you, there are many other strategies in this book to help you cope with your illness.

If you're in the third category, it may be worth taking some time to explore whether or not this could be an added source of support. For example, you might speak with a member of the clergy, discuss what you're going through, and ask how you might find spiritual support.

One final note: People who have always found solace in their spiritual beliefs might be shaken by the diagnosis of chronic illness. They may wonder why this could happen to them, and they may start questioning whether, in fact, there is a higher power. If you're looking to get back to a more comfortable spiritual level, consider meeting with a chaplain, spiritual counselor, or trusted guide to sort through questions and feelings. You might also ease back in by attending a service, joining a small group, or setting aside quiet time for prayer or reflection.

[ ] #155
Use Online Support Wisely

As we've discussed previously, the internet can be a very valuable resource. Not only can you gain a lot of helpful information, you can also gain support online.

How? There are moderated online support groups, chats, forums, blogs, webinars, and more, any of which can provide extra support and knowledge. The idea of finding a safe place online to talk about your diagnosis and get support from others with similar experiences can be very appealing. You just have to be careful, both in terms of what you hear from others, and whether or not any advice or leads you read about apply to you, and are safe for you.

As a result of all the potential benefits of the internet, it makes sense to spend a little time browsing. Start by doing a search of your illness, or any of the issues or questions you might have. Yes, you've done this before, in trying to learn about your condition. (See Strategy #24.) Here, focus on support-related communities and resources.

Once again, it's necessary to remind you (emphatically!) to use the internet wisely.

Make sure that any resources you check out are legitimate and make sense to you. Be critical and self-protective. Make sure the sites are reputable and respected. Don't give any personal information without confirming the site's credentials and privacy practices. Ask people in your network for advice on where to spend time. You'll find a link to a few of the safe, reliable websites that may be a helpful starting point.

To use this strategy:

In your Coping Notebook, start a page called "Online Support." List groups, organizations, or sites you're considering and note who runs them (patient organization, hospital, peer-run), whether they're moderated, and their privacy rules. Set a simple goal and limit (for example, "read/post 10–15 minutes, 3 times a week"). Protect your privacy (use a screen name; avoid sharing full name, address, or detailed medical data). Run medical tips by your clinician before acting on them, and discontinue going to sites that raise your stress level or you feel are counterproductive. Keep what helps; leave what doesn't.

[ ] #156

Use Technology for Self-Care

There are a number of valuable resources, materials, apps, or more that you can use to help your self-care efforts. For example, people who have smartphones may find it valuable to set reminders for important tasks, such as taking medication, calling the doctor for an appointment, implementing an exercise strategy, and tracking symptoms. There are apps for notes and reminders, relaxation, sleep, pain tracking, and nutrition.

Speak to others to find out how they have used technology to help them. Have fun checking out all of the possible types of technology that can help, but check reviews, costs, and privacy policies to confirm that the program, app or other resource you're considering is legitimate and cost-effective.

By and large, when you're overwhelmed with all the things you have to do, having valuable technological resources available can be very comforting. Just make sure they're safe. If a tool adds stress, it's not worth it.

To use this strategy:

Write a short "Tech Plan" in your Coping Notebook. Start with the problem you want help with (med reminders, sleep, pacing, mood). Pick one tool for one need and try it for two weeks. Turn on gentle reminders, keep notifications minimal, and review weekly: Is it helping? Is the data useful for you or your doctor? Keep what works, delete what doesn't, and add tools slowly so tech remains supportive, not overwhelming.

WHAT'S NEXT?

Your support system is one of your most valuable resources for coping with illness. By strengthening it, you reduce isolation and increase resilience. The next chapter will turn to practical ways to keep building your coping skills so you can continue moving forward with strength and confidence.

CHAPTER 10

I Need to Keep Moving Forward

This book has provided many strategies to help you cope, move forward, and reclaim your life with chronic illness. But your journey continues well beyond these pages. From here, the goal is simple: keep moving toward a happier, more meaningful life, even with your illness in the picture.

In this chapter, we'll add a few practical strategies to lean on when life gets bumpy, so you can keep feeling like yourself and keep doing what matters. Your Coping Notebook is your home base—jot down what you try, what helps, and what needs a tweak. When you feel stuck, use a quick double-column: on the left, what's hard or unclear; on the right, the next small step or the exact words you want to say. Let's keep going—at your pace, with tools that fit your life.

[ ] #157

Keep Asking What You Can Do Better *Today*

Small, specific actions build momentum. When progress feels slow, asking "what can I do better today?" keeps you moving and highlights progress you might overlook.

Think in terms of one doable improvement. You're not trying to fix everything—just to choose a clear next step that fits where you are today. Even tiny wins count. Each one helps practically and emotionally, and success fuels motivation.

Feeling better can bring impatience. If you catch yourself wanting everything to change at once, pause and bring the focus back to today's step. Whenever frustration shows up, ask, "What can I do right now?" Shift attention from the big picture to a single action you can take today.

Use your Coping Notebook to capture today's plan and to spot patterns over time. A quick weekly scan can show you how far you've come and what to adjust next so you stay motivated and see what's working.

To use this strategy:

Pick a consistent time—morning to set the day, or evening to plan for tomorrow—and open your Coping Notebook. Write one clear, realistic goal for the next 24 hours.

If a goal doesn't come to mind, skim your strategies and pick one area to nudge forward. If your thoughts feel vague, use a quick double-column to turn them into action: Left (Vague/Feeling): *I should exercise more.* → Right (Exact Step Today): Walk 10 minutes after lunch and jot down how I feel. Left (Worry): *I'm not improving fast enough.* → Right (Action): Text Jamie to drive me to Wednesday's 3:00 appointment; add it to the calendar.

Before setting tomorrow's goal, glance at today's note—what worked, what didn't, and one tweak. Keep goals bite-sized, check them off by day's end, and let the small wins add up.

[ ] #158

Anticipate and Conquer Obstacles

Obstacles are part of life after a diagnosis—that's normal. If/when an obstacle shows up, meet it then: name it, choose one small next step, and start dealing with it. You don't need the perfect fix—obstacles shrink one step at a time.

When something gets in your way, the goal is not perfection, it's movement. Name what's hard, pick from a few strategic options, and try one.

To use this strategy:

When you feel stuck, open your Coping Notebook and do a quick double-column to turn the obstacle into a plan. To guide you, ask yourself:

- What exactly is going on that has caused this block?
- What options are there to help you deal with this obstacle? (Consider strategies from this book, or other ideas you obtain from people you know.)
- What is your strategy-oriented plan to deal with the obstacle using the options that you have selected?

Be aware that you may encounter obstacles that you can't change. For those, your options should involve working on your thinking. You'll want to accept what is, deal with it as best you can, and focus your energy on things you can do something about.

[ ] #159

Take Good Care of Yourself

You are more than your illness. Good self-care blends what you have to do with what lifts your spirits, so your days feel balanced and you feel more like yourself. Keep the whole person in view—body, mind, relationships, and routines.

Taking good care of yourself is multifaceted. You want to prioritize both the things you have to do and the things you want to do. You want there to be a healthy balance of both in your life.

To use this strategy:

Open your Coping Notebook and sketch a simple two-column page— on the left, "Must-Do," on the right, "Want-To-Do." Take a minute to jot down what's already on your plate today, then add two or three things that would make the day feel more like you.

Now, instead of trying to do it all, gently pair the columns—one practical thing with one pleasant thing—so the day has a natural rhythm. For example, you might say, "Refill my prescription, and then call my friend Louise for ten minutes," or "Take a short walk, and later watch a TV episode I enjoy."

If energy dips or plans change, that's okay: circle the pair you can still manage, move the rest to tomorrow, and note how the pairing felt. The goal isn't perfection—it's a day that maximizes balance in your life.

[ ] #160

Identify Additional Problem Areas in Dealing with Your Illness

Many people diagnosed with a chronic illness share similar feelings early on, but each person's path evolves differently. To keep moving forward, it helps to identify those areas that are currently difficult for you.

The more precisely you can pinpoint your problem areas, the easier it will be to choose and apply strategies that fit.

Here are common areas that may be affected:

Family. Your family can be a great support. However, a diagnosis can affect everyone in your family. By being aware of how family members are affected, and helping them understand how you are affected, you can work more effectively together in coping with this change in life. Don't hesitate to seek guidance from trained professionals and reputable resources (books, support groups, trusted websites) for strategies to help you to deal with family relationships.

Relationships. Any significant relationships you are in can be affected by your diagnosis. You want your relationship to continue happily despite your diagnosis. As with family issues, there are many good strategies that you can use with your significant other.

On the other hand, if you are not currently in a relationship, it's common to worry about dating. People can and do meet potential partners despite a chronic illness. Keep your head high, be confident in yourself, and learn how to navigate any twists and turns.

Socialization. Your diagnosis may affect the social component of your life. This is especially possible if your symptoms make certain activities harder or energy is lower.

Friendships may change because of a chronic illness. You will learn who your true friends are—the ones who stick by you despite your diagnosis. Although it can be disappointing to see that some people who you thought were your friends move away from you, it's better to spend time with friends, current or new, who will be there to enjoy time with as you move forward with your life.

Activities. Your diagnosis may lead to changes in the things that you're able to do. It may have an impact on work, school, or leisure activities. Try not to dwell on what you can't do; focus on the things that you can do now or can learn to do, and build from there.

Work. Your diagnosis may affect your job. Clarify what you can do comfortably (your doctor can help). You'll want to figure out who to speak with at work, and decide what to share and when. You may also want to talk to your colleagues, to get them in the loop, so they can be more supportive.

School. If you're in school, symptoms may lead to missed days or slower progress. Talk with teachers about special accommodations and deadlines, and agree on a plan for any necessary adjustments. You'll also want to decide how much to discuss with your classmates, and what to say.

Emotions. At any point following your diagnosis, you may face feelings such as depression, sadness, anxiety, anger, guilt, boredom, or loneliness. Expect ups and downs. Be prepared for any emotional swings, and use supportive strategies to help you deal with them.

So, yes, there are a lot of things that you may face as you move forward following your diagnosis. This is just a brief overview. The good news is that there are things that can be done to help you deal with all of them. Learn about strategies to help you deal with your "hot spots". Some of the same strategies that you've read in this book can help you with these problem areas and can be a good start.

To use this strategy:

In your Coping Notebook, title a page, "Current Problem Areas". Indicate the areas that are current "hot spots" (family, relationships, social life, activities, work, school, emotions) and then circle the ones that are most important for you to handle. For each circled area, write one specific next step you can take this week and, if helpful, one person to involve. Revisit next week, note what helped, and pick the next small step to work on.

[ ] #161
Get Expert Advice About Financial Concerns

Once the initial shock of the diagnosis wears off, many people worry about the impact of their condition on their financial well-being. Professional guidance can lower stress and help you make clearer decisions.

There are many issues to consider: the cost of medication and other treatment components, costs of professional medical and ancillary care, insurance coverage, loss of earnings, and much more.

To use this strategy:

Since each person's situation is different, start by getting advice from people who work with cases like yours. That can include financial advisors, accountants, insurance agents, professionals who specialize in this area, and organizations that deal with these types of issues. There are plenty of people out there you can consult to start accumulating information that can help you deal with this issue.

In your Coping Notebook, keep a running list of questions (medication costs, coverage, disability options). Add names, contact information, and the answers you receive so you can compare options later.

[ ] #162

Benefit from Professional Assistance

There are dozens of strategies in this book, all designed to help you to answer, "Now what?", following your diagnosis. But any written book is trying to meet at least some needs for as many people as possible, so it couldn't perfectly cover all of the things that you may be going through in your life.

No matter how many strategies are included in this book, and no matter how many others could have been, there may still be times when you encounter a situation where you're not exactly sure what to do.

Some people find that they enjoy working on their strategies with a professional. This should be someone who works with those who have been diagnosed with a medical problem, but who can also learn about who you are, and specifically how you're affected, and help you implement strategies specifically for your needs.

If that's the case, there are many good professionals out there who can fill that role. Working with a professional can match the strategies you've read in this book to your needs. They can also offer tools you might not develop on your own.

To use this strategy:

In your Coping Notebook, note what kind of help you want (e.g., "manage anxiety before scans," "navigate insurance appeals"). List two or three professional options (therapist, medical social worker, patient navigator) and one question you'll ask each. After a first consultation, jot down what felt helpful and what you want to adjust so you can decide whether to continue or try for a better fit.

[ ] #163

Know When to Reread This Book

No, this wasn't a strategy designed to make you laugh. There may be times when you adjust to your diagnosis that you feel overwhelmed. You may just not understand why you're having a hard time. This is not uncommon, but it can be very upsetting.

That may be a good time to skim through this book again. Consider that there may be some very helpful strategies or things to think about that you've forgotten since you read them the first time. Or, maybe you read a strategy and, at that time, you did not see its relevance to you. Perhaps now things are different. It's possible your temporary roadblock can be helped with a previously unimplemented strategy.

It's worth reviewing the many strategies in this book to see what can help. Of course, even if the book doesn't have the answer, don't despair. That's a good time to reach out to someone on your support team to help you get moving again.

Naturally, there may be other reasons, besides having a hard time or encountering an obstacle, to reread this book. Look at it as a sensible strategy to keep it as an ongoing and available resource.

To use this strategy:

When you feel stuck or discouraged, open your Coping Notebook and write one line: "What's hard right now?" Then flip through the table of contents and select three strategies that might fit this current situation. Re-read those sections, pick one small step to try, and note the result. If nothing clicks, that's your cue to reach out to your support team.

*   *   *   *

What's Next?
Final Thoughts About
Moving Forward...

Our time together in these pages is ending, but your journey continues. You now have dozens of practical strategies to help you cope with your illness and keep moving forward—one clear step at a time.

Not every strategy will fit every day. Choose what helps now, adapt as your needs change, and remember that progress is built from many small, repeatable actions.

There will be ups and downs, and you are not powerless. Keep your Coping Notebook close. Capture what works, note questions for your care team, and lean on your support network. When things feel shaky, return to the strategies that helped before—let this book be a steady companion you can reopen whenever you want clarity, encouragement, or the next small step. Each day, ask: *What can I do right now to improve my life?*

Hold on to hope. New treatments and possibilities continue to emerge. Statistics are just numbers—there are always success stories. Why shouldn't one of them be yours?

Yes, you've been diagnosed. But you also have choices, strength, and resilience. This book was designed to help you cope, move forward, and reclaim your life. And as you progress, remember: No matter what problem you may face, you can always improve the quality of your life!

You can do this!

* * * *

Please note:

For updates, additional materials, announcements, and more, visit **www.coping.com/LWAD.**

Bookmark the website page and check back regularly—we'll share new information as it becomes available.

About the Author

Dr. Robert H. Phillips, founder and director of Long Island, NY's *Center for Coping* (**www.coping.com**), is a licensed psychologist who has been in private practice for more than 40 years and who has published and spoken widely on coping with physical ailments and other psychological topics. He has presented more than 500 papers and talks at seminars, conventions, and meetings throughout the United States and internationally. Dr. Phillips is on the national board of directors of the Autoimmune Association, has been on the national board of directors of the Lupus Foundation of America, and on medical advisory boards of, and the psychologist for, a number of major local and national organizations.

Dr. Phillips is also the author of more than 40 books, including *"Coping With Lupus"* (4th edition, Penguin Putnam/Avery, 2012), *"Lupus Q & A: Everything You Need To Know" (with Robert Lahita, MD)* (3rd edition, Penguin Putnam/Avery, 2014), " and *"Coping With Diabetes"* (Penguin Putnam/Avery, 2000). He is also the host of the popular "Coping Conversations" podcast (www.coping.com/podcast), interviewing celebrities and experts, available on all major podcast apps.